Longitudinal Research in Occupational Health Psychology

Occupational health psychology (OHP) involves the application of psychology to improving the quality of work life and to promoting and protecting the safety, health and well-being of employees. Achieving these aims requires researchers and practitioners to possess in-depth knowledge of the processes that are presumed to bring about the desired outcomes. To date, most studies in OHP have relied on cross-sectional designs in examining these processes. In such designs all variables of interest are measured simultaneously. Although this has generated many useful insights in how particular phenomena are associated, such designs cannot be trusted when it comes to drawing causal inferences: association is not causation.

This book therefore focuses on longitudinal research designs in OHP, whereby the concepts of interest are measured several times, offering much stronger evidence for causal relationships. The authors focus on design issues in longitudinal research (such as the number of measurements chosen, and the length of the time lags between these measurements), and illustrate these issues in the context of applied research on topics such as the work-family interface, conflict at work, and employee well-being. By doing so, this volume provides a state-of-the-art overview of current research in OHP, both in terms of its findings and methodologies.

This book is based on various special issues of the journal *Work & Stress*.

Toon W. Taris is Professor of Work and Organizational Psychology at Utrecht University, the Netherlands. He is currently Editor-in-Chief of *Work & Stress*. He has published extensively on topics such as longitudinal research methods, occupational health, stress, engagement, workaholism and authenticity at work.

Longitudinal Research in Occupational Health Psychology

Edited by
Toon W. Taris

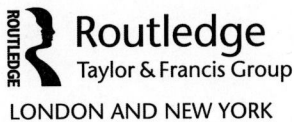

LONDON AND NEW YORK

First published 2016
by Routledge

2 Park Square, Milton Park, Abingdon, Oxon OX14 4RN
711 Third Avenue, New York, NY 10017, USA

Routledge is an imprint of the Taylor & Francis Group, an informa business

First issued in paperback 2017

British Library Cataloguing in Publication Data
A catalogue record for this book is available from the British Library

ISBN 13: 978-1-138-93346-0 (hbk)
ISBN 13: 978-1-138-09895-4 (pbk)

Typeset in Times New Roman
by RefineCatch Limited, Bungay, Suffolk

Publisher's Note
The publisher accepts responsibility for any inconsistencies that may have
arisen during the conversion of this book from journal articles to book chapters,
namely the possible inclusion of journal terminology.

Disclaimer
Every effort has been made to contact copyright holders for their permission to
reprint material in this book. The publishers would be grateful to hear from any
copyright holder who is not here acknowledged and will undertake to rectify
any errors or omissions in future editions of this book.

Contents

CONTENTS

Citation Information

The chapters in this book were originally published in various special issues of the journal *Work & Stress*. When citing this material, please use the original volume and issue information and page numbering for each article, as follows:

Chapter 1
Editorial: Cause and effect: Optimizing the designs of longitudinal studies in occupational health psychology
Toon W. Taris and Michiel A.J. Kompier
Work & Stress, volume 28, issue 1 (January–March 2014) pp. 1–8

Chapter 2
How do occupational stressor-strain effects vary with time? A review and meta-analysis of the relevance of time lags in longitudinal studies
Michael T. Ford, Russell A. Matthews, Jessica D. Wooldridge, Vipanchi Mishra, Urszula M. Kakar and Sarah R. Strahan
Work & Stress, volume 28, issue 1 (January–March 2014) pp. 9–30

Chapter 3
The effect of conflict at work on well-being: Depressive symptoms as a vulnerability factor
Laurenz L. Meier, Norbert K. Semmer and Sven Gross
Work & Stress, volume 28, issue 1 (January–March 2014) pp. 31–48

Chapter 4
Enjoyment and absorption: An electronic diary study on daily flow patterns
Alma M. Rodríguez-Sánchez, Wilmar Schaufeli, Marisa Salanova, Eva Cifre and Mieke Sonnenschein
Work & Stress, volume 25, issue 1 (January–March 2011) pp. 75–92

Chapter 5
Effects of vacation from work on health and well-being: Lots of fun, quickly gone
Jessica de Bloom, Sabine A.E. Geurts, Toon W. Taris, Sabine Sonnentag, Carolina de Weerth and Michiel A.J. Kompier
Work & Stress, volume 24, issue 2 (April–June 2010) pp. 196–216

Chapter 6

Work to non-work enrichment: The mediating roles of positive affect and positive work reflection
Stefanie Daniel and Sabine Sonnentag
Work & Stress, volume 28, issue 1 (January–March 2014) pp. 49–66

Chapter 7

Do you want me to be perfect? Two longitudinal studies on socially prescribed perfectionism, stress and burnout in the workplace
Julian H. Childs and Joachim Stoeber
Work & Stress, volume 26, issue 4 (October–December 2012) pp. 347–364

Chapter 8

A participative intervention to improve employee well-being in knowledge work jobs: A mixed-methods evaluation study
Ole Henning Sørensen and David Holman
Work & Stress, volume 28, issue 1 (January–March 2014) pp. 67–86

Chapter 9

Should I stay or should I go? Examining longitudinal relations among job resources and work engagement for stayers versus movers
Annet H. de Lange, Hans De Witte and Guy Notelaers
Work & Stress, volume 22, issue 3 (July–September 2008) pp. 201–223

Chapter 10

Are job and personal resources associated with work ability 10 years later? The mediating role of work engagement
Auli Airila, Jari J. Hakanen, Wilmar B. Schaufeli, Ritva Luukkonen, Anne Punakallio and Sirpa Lusa
Work & Stress, volume 28, issue 1 (January–March 2014) pp. 87–105

For any permission-related enquiries please visit:
http://www.tandfonline.com/page/help/permissions

Cause and effect: Optimizing the designs of longitudinal studies in occupational health psychology

According to the National Institute for Occupational Safety and Health, occupational health psychology (OHP) involves "the application of psychology to improving the quality of work life, and to protecting and promoting the safety, health and well-being of workers" (NIOSH, 2013). Although not everyone may agree with this definition (is OHP-research only about the *application* of currently available psychological knowledge to working life, or does it also *generate* new and even fundamental insights?), to make a difference in workers' lives is certainly a key concern in our discipline. Achieving this aim requires in-depth knowledge of the causal processes that affect these desiderata: healthy work and healthy workers. In order to obtain such knowledge, we need longitudinal studies in which the same variables are measured at least twice across time for the same set of participants (e.g. Hassett & Paavilainen-Mäntymäki, 2013; Menard, 2007; Ployhart & Vandenberg, 2010). Although cross-sectional designs can tell us whether particular variables are associated in ways that are proposed by theories, longitudinal research designs can also provide us with information about the temporal order of the events underlying these associations, show how the presumed "outcomes" have changed across time and whether this change can be ascribed to (changes in) the alleged "independent" variables. Accordingly, over the last two decades the number of OHP studies examining causal processes through longitudinal research designs has increased steadily (see, for instance, Austin, Scherbaum, & Mahlmann, 2002; Stone-Romero, 2011). A number of such studies are included in this special edition of *Work & Stress*, which is devoted to longitudinal research.

An intriguing question is whether our *understanding* of the causal underpinnings of occupational safety, health and well-being has increased at a similar pace. To some extent it has: longitudinal studies have often confirmed and clarified relations that were previously mainly obtained in cross-sectional research. For example, by now we know that high job demands, low support and low control adversely affect well-being longitudinally and, by implication, causally (Häusser, Mojzisch, Niesel, & Schulz-Hardt, 2010). However, longitudinal studies have also produced unexpected and confusing findings, and sometimes have not replicated associations that had been firmly established cross-sectionally. We believe that this is at least partly due to poor *a priori* consideration of what exactly should be the right longitudinal design for studying the specific causal relations at hand. That is, researchers should carefully consider their choice of research design in the light of theories on the specific relations under study, previous empirical studies on these relations, and practical considerations, paying due attention to each of these three aspects. In this editorial we focus on two pivotal sets of issues that warrant more attention, namely (1) the length of the time intervals employed in longitudinal designs, and (2) the issue of reciprocal (i.e. bi-directional) effects.

Time lags in longitudinal designs

The appropriate length of the time lags between study waves is a crucial issue in longitudinal research methodology. The length of this interval should correspond well with the underlying "true" causal lag (e.g. De Lange, Taris, Kompier, Houtman, & Bongers, 2004; Dormann & Zapf, 2002; Ployhart & Vandenberg, 2010; Zapf, Dormann, & Frese, 1996). If it is much shorter than the true causal lag, chances are that the antecedent has not yet had sufficient time to affect the outcome variable. Conversely, if this interval is too long, the effect of being exposed to the antecedent variable may already have disappeared. To complicate things further, in the intervening period between study waves all kinds of other events may take place that compete with the Time 1 exposure in affecting the outcome variables. Such competing factors may affect the internal validity of the study in that the strength of the effect between predictor and effect will be biased downwards. Further, employees are not just passive recipients of situational stimuli, but may try to change their work situation. Between the study waves, they may, for example, try to change their job content, working conditions or working time arrangements (Wrzesniewski & Dutton, 2001). When time intervals are too short or too long, the chances of detecting the effects of the antecedent variable on the outcome will decrease, as compared to when the study interval corresponds with the true underlying interval. All this implies that (1) the magnitude of the longitudinal effects may vary strongly with the length of the interval used, and (2) that to advance longitudinal research, scholars should carefully consider the possible underlying causal time lags before they conduct their study. When this true time lag is unknown or cannot be reasonably surmised, researchers should preferably employ multiphase designs in which measurements are taken from the same set of participants at several points in time (Ployhart & Vandenberg, 2010; Taris & Kompier, 2003), the lengths of the intervals between measurements being appropriate to the variables under study. We believe that these recommendations are appropriate because as yet the number of study waves and the length of the interval between these waves is often chosen on pragmatic grounds.

Despite the increase in longitudinal studies, to date the two-wave longitudinal design has continued to dominate the research scene, with the possible exception of the diary study (Bolger, Davis, & Rafaeli, 2003). Diary studies tend to focus on relatively volatile processes in which the phenomena of interest (e.g. mood or fatigue) change quickly over time. Typically, a relatively small number of participants completes short questionnaires repeatedly during the day, on a number of consecutive days. Due to this repeated measures design, within-participant changes in the phenomena of interest can be related to the "little experiences of everyday life" that precede these changes (Wheeler & Reis, 1991, p. 340). Similarly, spill-over effects from one day to another can be examined, for example, from working days to a non-work day. Unfortunately, the potential benefits of the diary design in examining causal processes are not always realized. Establishing temporal order requires that the outcome variable (e.g. well-being) is related not only to a particular predictor (e.g. recovery experiences) as measured earlier that day or on the previous day, but also to well-being as measured earlier (e.g. on the previous day). If this requirement is not met, diary designs are not more informative regarding the development of causal processes than a purely cross-sectional approach (Kelloway & Francis, 2013).

At present, when the research focus is not on explaining changes in day-to-day experiences, the two-wave longitudinal design remains the most frequently used approach. Thus, the choice of a particular interval between the study waves becomes paramount. Dormann and Zapf (2002) and De Lange et al. (2004) conducted studies using multi-wave longitudinal designs in order to examine how the strength of the effects in longitudinal research depended on the length of the interval between the study waves. Dormann and Zapf (2002), comparing findings over one-year, two-year and four-year intervals, found that it took at least two years for the longitudinal effects of stressors at work on mental health (measured as depressive symptoms mediated by irritation) to be demonstrated and that they were weakest at one year. Similarly, De Lange et al. (2004), using time lags of one, two and three years, reported that the longitudinal effects between job stressors and health (depression, emotional exhaustion and job satisfaction) were strongest for a one-year interval. By the end of 2013 these two studies had jointly received nearly 500 citations, but in the light of the above discussion their value as a *general* foundation for the choice for a particular time interval is limited. Not only do their findings regarding the optimal interval between the study waves differ, but it is also likely that their findings do not generalize beyond the type of stressors and outcomes studied. This reasoning follows from a seminal study by Frese and Zapf (1994) who distinguished among five types of developmental trajectories for the processes typically studied in OHP. For example, workers may get used to some stressors quickly, meaning that the effects of exposure to these stressors may be short-lived and that a short interval between the study waves is required to detect these effects. Other work factors may affect health only in the long run, and are referred to by Ford et al. (2014) in the first paper in this special edition of *Work & Stress* as lagged effects. Clearly, simple general rules of thumb regarding the appropriate length of the time interval for a study do not exist. This implies that any sensible choice for a particular time interval between the study waves must necessarily take into account the type of causes and consequences being investigated, as well as consider the development and context of the process that is being examined.

Reciprocal effects

Normal and reversed effects constitute another issue in longitudinal research. In a previous editorial on longitudinal designs (Taris & Kompier, 2003) we recommended researchers to more often employ full panel designs: designs in which both the presumed "outcomes" and "explanatory" variables are assessed at all study waves. We believe that, over the last decade, one of the strong developments in OHP has been the increase in the number of studies employing these designs. Full panel designs allow for the examination of both normal and reversed effects. *Normal effects* usually refer to the lagged effects of job characteristics on safety, health, well-being and performance-related variables. *Reversed effects* relate to effects of the latter categories of variables on job characteristics. Inspired by the seminal work of Zapf et al. (1996), De Lange et al. (2004) discussed a number of mechanisms that could account for reversed effects. They argued that there are multiple reasons why employees who report high levels of ill health at Time 1 could report higher levels of job demands at Time 2. For example, such employees (assuming that their coping capacity is limited) may only *perceive* their jobs as having become more demanding (i.e. the demands themselves did not change). It is also possible that ill health causes a "drift" towards an objectively more demanding job (see, for instance, Kompier & Taris, 2011, for a discussion). When a study supports both normal and reversed effects, researchers speak of *reciprocal* effects.

The increase in the number of longitudinal studies in OHP during the last decade went hand in hand with a more frequent examination of possible reversed and reciprocal effects (among others, De Jonge et al., 2001; De Lange et al., 2004; Rodriguez-Munoz, Sanz-Vergel, Demerouti, & Bakker, 2012). In itself this is a positive development. A strong example is a study by Finne, Knardahl, and Lau (2011) on workplace bullying and mental distress. Whereas self-reported workplace bullying predicted mental distress two years later (signifying normal causation), mental distress also predicted bullying across time (indicating reverse causation). Apparently, the associations between workplace bullying and mental distress constitute a vicious circle, with bullying leading to mental problems and the latter leading to higher levels of bullying, and so forth. However, such exemplary studies notwithstanding, as yet we do lack a more systematic integration of such effects into OHP theory, i.e. into the body of knowledge on the processes relating work characteristics to worker health, well-being, safety and performance. Currently a fairly impressionistic picture of these reversed/reciprocal effects emerges: sometimes such effects are absent, sometimes present (and in that case researchers are happy to report and interpret them), but we are still in need of a more *integrated theory* that describes (1) *when* and (2) *what sort of effects* can be expected (3) *for whom* in (4) *which circumstances* and (5) what the *specific processes* responsible for such effects could be. We might add that even the terms "normal" versus "reversed" effects themselves are problematic: What is normal about "normal" causality? This label derives from the fact that researchers "normally" examine the effects of work stressors on strains, rather than that it reflects a characteristic of these effects themselves. Consequently, it might be more accurate to speak of "stressor-to-strain effects" instead of normal causality, and of "strain-to-stressor effects" in the instance of reversed effects.

Another notable exception to the above observation that longitudinal studies have served to clarify the causal processes underlying occupational safety, health and well-being concerns the body of research on *gain and loss spirals* in OHP. Building on Fredrickson's (2001) broaden-and-build theory of positive emotions, through longitudinal research it has been found that the presence of job resources (such as high levels of autonomy and support) tends to promote well-being (such as high levels of work engagement) over time, and that high levels of engagement in turn lead to high levels of job resources (see Salanova, Schaufeli, Xanthopoulou, & Bakker, 2010, for an overview). This research suggests that engaged workers tend to collect more resources in their job, leading to even higher levels of engagement (the so-called gain spiral), whereas low-engagement workers tend to lose job resources, leading to even lower levels of engagement (the loss spiral). In spite of such well-demonstrated longitudinal reciprocal effects, it is not entirely clear how a gain (or loss) spiral would develop in practice, especially since deprived workers may attempt to improve the quality of their jobs (Wrzesniewski & Dutton, 2001), and supervisors and colleagues may see to it that any resources available are distributed equitably across all workers. Indeed, one might even question whether such cycles have actually been demonstrated. Gain and loss cycles refer to changes in the *levels* of engagement and resources, but the evidence available today draws on correlational (regression) analyses. Correlations show how strongly the *relative order* of the scores of participants on one variable corresponds with the order of their scores on other variables. Strong correlations indicate that participants whose scores on one variable are relatively high, usually obtain relatively high (or low) scores on other variables as well. That is, the order of participants is either largely the same (in the case of strong positive correlations) or largely the reverse (for strong negative correlations) across variables. However, information on the correspondence of the relative order of the scores of the participants on the study variables tells us nothing about the stability or change in terms of the level of these variables: strong correlations may coincide with increases, decreases, or no change at all in the levels of the respective variables (see Mortimer, Finch & Kumka, 1982, for a discussion). Since the current evidence is almost exclusively based on correlations, it cannot support any claims regarding the existence of gain and loss cycles, as these refer to changes in the *levels* of engagement and resources. In order to examine such cycles properly, we should examine the across-time development of mean levels of engagement (and resources) for low- and high-resources (engagement) groups (see, for instance, Salanova et al., 2010), rather than look only at suggestive – but irrelevant – patterns of lagged correlation or regression estimates. Thus, it appears that even in the case of this theoretically relatively well-developed field of research, where stressor-to-strain and strain-to-stressor effects are vitally important and have received considerable attention, scholars have given insufficient attention to the optimization of the design and analysis of their studies.

Implications

What does all this mean for research in the area of occupational health psychology? First and foremost, before conducting a longitudinal study, researchers should *think about their study design*. Although such designs are much more useful for establishing causal relationships than cross-sectional designs, they are no panacea and could yield disappointing and even misleading findings (e.g. when failing to detect an effect that is present in the population). One of the most important issues is the length of the interval between two consecutive study waves: this should correspond as closely as possible with the true, underlying causal interval between stressor and strain. Researchers should consider this issue thoroughly in the design phase of their study, not only considering pragmatic issues, but certainly also taking into account theories on the specific relations under study and previous empirical studies on these relations.

Secondly, we also encourage researchers to explicitly *report their reasons for choosing a particular time interval*. The choice of interval between the study waves can be considered the practical translation of a hypothesis on how one variable affects another. In this sense, it should not be too much to ask researchers to provide an explicit justification for this hypothesis: that is, why is this particular interval appropriate, given the variables and processes under study? Stated differently, we propose that the choice of a particular time interval should be part of the theoretical foundation of a study since it should be based on a researcher's theory on how variables affect each other: it is certainly not solely a matter of convenience or practical possibilities. In the absence of solid grounds for choosing a particular time interval between the study waves, we recommend that researchers *include multiple waves in their design*, with relatively short time intervals between these waves. Exactly how short will depend on the nature of the variables under study. In this way they would maximize the chances of including the "right" interval between the study waves.

Thirdly, researchers are to be commended for recognizing that a particular association between two variables can be due to both stressor-to-strain and strain-to-stressor processes. However, the next step – systematically incorporating findings on reciprocal causation into their theories – has as yet not been taken. Researchers should by all means employ full panel designs to test reciprocal stressor-to-strain and strain-to-stressor effects. However, we also encourage them to *indicate more clearly what the scientific and practical added value of doing so could be*, and to *develop their designs in such a way that they can actually test the predictions of their theories on reciprocal causation*. To date there is some evidence for processes in which variables mutually influence each other, but this does not appear to have led to an integrated theory on how work characteristics and work outcomes reciprocally affect each other. In the absence of such a theory, it is difficult to appreciate the added value of examining reciprocal effects. Thus, researchers should not only test for such effects, they should also think about the implications of their findings, both with regard to the specific issue under study and in the context of the broader area of occupational health psychology.

The present special issue: Longitudinal research in occupational health psychology

Longitudinal designs offer substantial advantages over cross-sectional designs in examining causal processes in occupational health psychology. Since the beginning of this century the number of longitudinal studies in OHP has increased, constituting a major step forward in our field. Further, journals have become increasingly reluctant to publish cross-sectional studies, and the quality of the longitudinal designs used in OHP has improved. Another positive development is a stronger focus on the potential bi-directional relations between work factors and indicators of worker health and well-being. On the other hand, researchers should not routinely opt for a full panel design with only two study waves, and forget to pay full attention to what would theoretically be the optimal time interval "for things to happen" in their study. Also, they should aim to further develop theory on how reverse causation effects can be explained. All in all, we believe that researchers can only get the best out of studies having longitudinal designs if they consider the strengths and pitfalls of these designs more thoroughly than is too often currently the case.

The current issue of *Work & Stress* starts off with an excellent review by Michael Ford et al. (2014) that addresses these issues. Drawing on a review and meta-analysis of 68 longitudinal studies, they examine (1) the extent to which correlations between stressors and strains when both are measured at the same time point (i.e. *synchronous* effects) change with the passage of time, and (2) the extent to which stressors longitudinally predict increases in strain (i.e. *lagged* effects) and how these effects vary across different time lags. Their results show that *synchronous* effects of chronic stressors tend to increase over time, and that the strength of the *lagged* association between work stressors and strains peaks at, on average, three years after the first study wave. They further examine this issue as a function of different types of outcome, and also address the subject of reciprocal effects.

In conjunction, the other contributions to this special issue provide an interesting overview of longitudinal designs as they are commonly used in occupational health psychology. In the first of these contributions, Meier, Semmer, and Gross (2014) present two associated studies on the effects of conflict at work. Whereas the first employs a cross-sectional design, the second is a two-week diary study. In conjunction, these studies suggest that conflict may lead to depressive symptoms, and that these in turn make people even more vulnerable to conflict.

In the next paper, Daniel and Sonnentag (2014) present a two-wave, three-month study on engagement and work-life balance, showing that positive affect and reflection on the positive aspects of work during leisure time mediated the relationship between work engagement and work-to-life enrichment. They argue that such enrichment should in turn benefit the employer. Sorensen and Holman (2014) conducted an elaborate, mixed-methods participative intervention study that included both a qualitative and quantitative evaluation. The qualitative evaluation employed a pre/post-test design, with a 10-month interval between the two waves. The study showed that the intervention yielded significant improvements in burnout and workers' relationships with their supervisor and colleagues. Finally in this edition, Airila et al. (2014) examine the relations between personal resources and work ability in a two-wave, 10-year longitudinal study. In spite of this very long time interval, their study provided indications that job engagement mediates the relationship between job and personal resources, and workability.

We believe that these studies all present important additions to knowledge on the associations between work and personal characteristics on the one hand, and health and well-being on the other, and that this is in a large part due to the fact that the authors of these papers make the most out of the longitudinal designs underlying their research.

References

Airila, A., Hakanen, J., Schaufeli, W. B., Luukkonen, R., Punakallio, A., & Lusa, S. (2014). Are job and personal resources associated with work ability 10 years later? The mediating role of work engagement. *Work & Stress, 28*, 87–105.

Austin, J. T., Scherbaum, C. A., & Mahlman, R. A. (2002). History of research methods in industrial and organizational psychology: Measurement, design, analysis. In S. G. Rogelberg (Ed.), *Handbook of research methods in industrial and organizational psychology* (pp. 3–33). Malden: Blackwell.

Bolger, N., Davis, A., & Rafaeli, E. (2003). Diary methods: Capturing life as it is lived. *Annual Review of Psychology, 54*, 579–616.

Daniel, S., & Sonnentag, S. (2014). Work to non-work enrichment: The mediating roles of positive affect and positive work reflection. *Work & Stress, 28*, 49–66.

De Jonge, J., Dormann, C., Janssen, P. P. M., Dollard, M. F., Landeweerd, J. A., & Nijhuis, F. J. N. (2001). Testing reciprocal relationships between job characteristics and psychological well-being: A cross-lagged structural equation analysis. *Journal of Occupational and Organizational Psychology, 74*, 29–45.

De Lange, A. H., Taris, T. W., Kompier, M. A. J., Houtman, I. L. D., & Bongers, P. M. (2004). The relationships between work characteristics and mental health: Examining normal, reversed and reciprocal relationships in a 4-wave study. *Work & Stress, 18*(2), 149–166.

Dormann, C., & Zapf, D. (2002). Social stressors at work, irritation, and depressive symptoms: Accounting for unmeasured third variables in a multi-wave study. *Journal of Occupational and Organizational Psychology, 75*(1), 33–58.

Finne, L. B., Knardahl, S., & Lau, B. (2011). Workplace bullying and mental distress. A prospective study of Norwegian employees. *Scandinavian Journal of Work, Environment and Health, 37*(4), 276–287.

Ford, M., Matthews, R., Wooldridge, J., Vipanchi, M., Kakar, U., & Strahan, S. (2014). How do occupational stressor-strain effects vary with time? A review and meta-analysis of the relevance of time lags in longitudinal studies. *Work & Stress, 28*, 9–30.

Fredrickson, B. L. (2001). The role of positive emotions in positive psychology. *American Psychologist, 56*, 218–226.

Frese, M., & Zapf, D. (1994). Methodological issues in the study of work stress: Objective vs subjective measurement of work stress and the question of longitudinal studies. In C. L. Cooper & R. Payne (Eds.), *Causes, coping and consequences of stress at work* (pp. 375–411). Chichester: Wiley.

Hassett, M., & Paavilainen-Mäntymäki, E. (Eds.). (2013). *Handbook of longitudinal research methods in organisation and business studies*. London: Edward Elgar.

Häusser, J. A., Mojzisch, A., Niesel, M., & Schulz-Hardt, S. (2010). Ten years on: A review of recent research on the Job Demand-Control (-Support) model and psychological well-being. *Work & Stress, 24*(1), 1–35.

Kelloway, E. K., & Francis, L. (2013). Longitudinal research and longitudinal data analysis. In R. R. Sinclair, M. Wang, & L. E. Tetrick (Eds.), *Research methods in occupational health psychology* (pp. 374–394). New York, NY: Routledge.

Kompier, M. A. J., & Taris, T. W. (2011). Understanding the causal relations between psychosocial factors at work and health: A circular process. *Scandinavian Journal of Work, Environment, and Health, 37*, 259–261.

Meier, L., Semmer, N., & Gross, S. (2014). The effect of conflict at work on well-being: Depressive symptoms as a vulnerability factor. *Work & Stress, 28*, 31–48.

Menard, S. (Ed.). (2007). *Handbook of longitudinal design: Design, measurement and analysis*. New York, NY: Academic Press.

Mortimer, J. T., Finch, M. D., & Kumka, D. (1982). Persistence and change in development: The multidimensional self-concept. In P. B. Baltes & O. G. Brim, Jr. (Eds.), *Life span development and behavior* (Vol. 4, pp. 263–313). New York, NY: Academic Press.

National Institute for Occupational Safety and Health (NIOSH). (2013). *What is OHP?* Retrieved December 5, 2013, from http://www.cdc.gov/niosh/topics/ohp/#what.

Ployhart, R. E., & Vandenberg, R. J. (2010). Longitudinal research: The theory, design, and analysis of change. *Journal of Management, 36*(1), 94–120.

Rodriguez-Munoz, A., Sanz-Vergel, A. I., Demerouti, E., & Bakker, A. B. (2012). Reciprocal relationships between job demands, job resources, and recovery opportunities. *Journal of Personnel Psychology, 11*(2), 86–94.

Salanova, M., Schaufeli, W. B., Xanthopoulou, D., & Bakker, A. B. (2010). The gain spiral of resources and work engagement: Sustaining a positive worklife. In A. B. Bakker & M. P. Leiter (Eds.), *Work engagement: A handbook of essential theory and research* (pp. 118–131). New York, NY: Psychology Press.

Sorensen, O., & Holman, D. (2014). A participative intervention to improve employee well-being in knowledge work jobs: A mixed-methods evaluation study. *Work & Stress, 28*, 67–86.

Stone-Romero, E. (2011). Research strategies in industrial and organizational psychology: Nonexperimental, quasi-experimental, and randomized experimental research in special purpose and nonspecial purpose settings. In S. Zedeck (Ed.), *APA Handbook of industrial and organizational psychology, Vol. 1: Building and developing the organization* (pp. 37–72). Washington, DC: American Psychological Association.

Taris, T. W., & Kompier, M. A. J. (2003). Challenges in longitudinal designs in occupational health psychology. *Scandinavian Journal of Work, Environment and Health, 29*, 1–4.

Wheeler, L., & Reis, H. T. (1991). Self-recording of everyday life events: Origins, types, and uses. *Journal of Personality, 59*, 339–354.

Wrzesniewski, A., & Dutton, J. E. (2001). Crafting a job: Revisioning employees as active crafters of their work. *Academy of Management Review, 26*, 179–201.

Zapf, D., Dormann, C., & Frese, M. (1996). Longitudinal studies in organizational stress research: A review of the literature with reference to methodological issues. *Journal of Occupational Health Psychology, 1*(2), 145–169.

Toon W. Taris, Editor, *Work & Stress*
Department of Social and Organizational Psychology,
Utrecht University, The Netherlands

Michiel A. J. Kompier
Behavioural Science Institute, Radboud University Nijmegen,
The Netherlands

How do occupational stressor-strain effects vary with time? A review and meta-analysis of the relevance of time lags in longitudinal studies

Michael T. Ford[a], Russell A. Matthews[b], Jessica D. Wooldridge[a], Vipanchi Mishra[c], Urszula M. Kakar[d] and Sarah R. Strahan[a]

[a]Department of Psychology, University at Albany, SUNY, Albany, NY, USA; [b]Department of Psychology, Bowling Green State University, Bowling Green, OH, USA; [c]Department of Psychology, Iona College, New Rochelle NY, USA; [d]City and County of San Francisco, San Francisco, CA, USA

Through a meta-analysis of longitudinal studies from 68 samples, this study examines the role of time in three types of occupational stressor-strain effects. First, this study reviews the extent to which correlations between stressors and strains when both are measured at the same time point (i.e. *synchronous* effects) change with the passage of time. Second, this review examines the extent to which stressors predict increases in strain (i.e. *lagged* effects) and whether these effects vary across different time lags. Third, this paper considers the extent to which strains predict increases in stressors (i.e. *reverse causation* effects), and whether these effects vary across different time lags. Results indicate that synchronous effects tend to increase over time, suggesting that the effects of chronic stressors build up through cumulative exposure. Lagged effects were generally small but their magnitude increased over time for about three years before declining, whereas the average size of reverse causation effects was also small but tended to increase across time. The lagged and reverse causation effects were highly variable, especially among studies with sample sizes under 500, suggesting that large sample sizes are needed to detect them reliably. Implications for longitudinal occupational stress theory and research are discussed.

Introduction

In the organizational sciences there has been a burgeoning interest in the role of time in organizationally-relevant variables (Mitchell & James, 2001). One topic in organizational research where the passage of time is paramount is the association between chronic workplace stressors (i.e. working conditions that are indefinite in duration) and employee psychological and physical well-being (i.e. strain). It is often stated that longitudinal designs are preferable to cross-sectional designs in organizational research because the research questions usually involve change. Longitudinal designs are seen as the best way to address such questions about change (Bono & McNamara, 2011). Despite this emphasis on longitudinal research, surprisingly little is known about how workplace stressor-strain relations vary across time and the accompanying theoretical implications. Perhaps equally important, it is not clear how reliable or consistent the results have been in longitudinal stress research and the sample sizes needed for reasonable power to detect such effects. In this manuscript, we inductively examine these issues by quantitatively reviewing longitudinal research on occupational stressor-strain relations and discussing the theoretical and methodological implications of the pattern of results across studies. This is the first quantitative review of these effects to our knowledge.

Placed within a temporal theoretical framework, the empirically observed effects of chronic workplace stressors on strain take two forms. The first form is the *synchronous* effect or short-term reaction. Synchronous effects are concurrent, such that higher stressor levels are associated with strain at the same point in time. For example, an increase in work overload may cause a worker to experience an increase in fatigue immediately or within a day or two. This elevated fatigue level may last until the workload is reduced, after which the fatigue level quickly decreases until the workload increases again. These reactions develop relatively immediately and are observed via within-time-period or cross-sectional correlations. The second type of observed effect is the *lagged* effect, which occurs when the effect of a stressor takes time to develop. For example, a worker may first respond resiliently to heavy workload and show little or no change in fatigue. However, there may be a delayed reaction such that fatigue increases at a later point in time. This lagged effect, sometimes called the "sleeper" effect (Garst, Frese, & Molenaar, 2000), is operationalized as the extent to which a stressor at one point in time predicts strains at a later point in time, controlling for baseline strain levels. In conjunction with synchronous and lagged effects is a related *reverse causation* effect. The reverse causation effect is operationalized as the extent to which strains at one point in time predict stressors at a later point in time, controlling for baseline stressor levels. For example, a worker with poor psychological health may suffer from poorer performance, and as a result experience an unfavourable change in working conditions involving an increase in stressors. This change in stressors is likely to take some time and thus result in a lagged strain-to-stressor effect.

If a researcher measures workload and psychological well-being at one point in time and then measures these same two variables one year later, each of these three types of stressor-strain effect can be estimated. First, the correlation between workload at Time 1 and psychological well-being at Time 1 would represent a synchronous effect, as would the correlation between workload at Time 2 and psychological well-being at Time 2. Second, the lagged effect would be represented by the effect of Time 1 workload on Time 2 psychological well-being, controlling for Time 1 psychological well-being in a regression model. Finally, the reverse causation effect would be represented by the effect of Time 1 psychological well-being on Time 2 workload, controlling for Time 1 workload in a regression model.

The literature on the role of time in synchronous, lagged or reverse causation effects among chronic occupational stressors and strains is currently limited in two notable ways. First, there has been little attention given to how synchronous effects develop over time. At any point in time a cross-sectional or synchronous correlation between stressors and strains may be computed. If assessed at a later point in time, will this correlation tend to increase, decrease or stay the same, holding other variables equal? We propose – based on theoretical views on cumulative resource depletion and allostatic load – that synchronous effects tend to strengthen over time. Second, there is little empirically-based guidance on appropriate time frames for lagged and reverse causation effects. Indeed, de Lange, Taris, Kompier, Houtman, and Bongers (2003) noted in their review article that researchers have limited resources available for setting time lags in multi-wave longitudinal studies on occupational stress, and that, of the information that is available for setting appropriate time lags between measurements in panel studies of stressors and strains, much of it seems unclear or speculative. In this paper we address each of these issues through a review and analysis of relevant longitudinal studies.

Occupational stressors and strain

Occupational stressors are conditions and events in the work environment that bring about strain (Kahn & Byosiere, 1992). Although some occupational stressors are the result of discrete traumatic experiences (e.g. a workplace shooting) or change processes (e.g. business reorganization), most are a function of chronic working conditions that are indefinite in duration. Sonnentag and Frese (2003), in their review of occupational stress research, identified five types of chronic stressors that reflect these chronic working conditions: physical stressors, task-related stressors, role stressors, social stressors and schedule-related stressors. In this study, we incorporate all but schedule-related stressors, which are more applicable to some work populations than to others and therefore may not yield comparable effects across samples.

Strains can be psychological or physical. Psychological strains generally refer to stable negative affective and cognitive states that emerge in response to stressors that are perceived to tax or exceed the worker's resources (Hobfoll, 1989; Lazarus & Folkman, 1984). We structure these negative states by using the negative half of Russell's (1980) affective circumplex, which includes three types of strains: high-arousal strains such as anxiety and irritation, low-arousal strains such as depression and exhaustion, and general negative psychological well-being. Common physical stress reactions include psychosomatic complaints such as headaches, colds, fevers, dizziness and gastrointestinal problems (Spector & Jex, 1998). These have been found to be associated with various types of chronic stressors (Nixon, Mazzola, Bauer, Krueger, & Spector, 2011).

It is particularly important to distinguish the different types of strain in analyses of longitudinal occupational stress effects because the time course of these effects may differ across the types of strain. For example, physical strains may take longer to develop because they require some cumulative wear and tear on the body. In contrast, anxiety, being more proximal to the perception of the stressors, may occur more immediately. These potential differences are discussed in more detail below and are tested for in this analysis.

Changes in synchronous stress reactions

Synchronous stressor-strain effects are the result of a concurrent association between stressors and strains. This association occurs to the extent that increases/decreases in stressor levels are accompanied by concurrent increases/decreases in strains. Synchronous stressor-strain effects are observed as cross-sectional correlations. Field research suggests that stressor-strain associations can develop fairly quickly. For example, in one of the few job stress studies to sample workers as they first began employment, school teachers who entered low-stressor positions differed little from those entering high-stressor positions in their level of strain upon entry. However, after four months those in high-stressor positions reported much higher depression and physical symptom levels (Schonfeld, 1996), suggesting that strains develop in four months or less after initial exposure to chronic stressors. Conversely, there is evidence that much of the effect of stressors on strains fades away quickly when chronic stressors are removed. For example, Westman and Eden (1997) found that the synchronous correlation between workplace stressors and burnout declined substantially (from $r = .63$ to .22) during a vacation, suggesting strains diminish quickly as stressors are removed. Frese and Zapf (1988) developed what they termed the "initial impact model" to describe these short-term, synchronous reactions. According to this model, there is an immediate strain reaction to workplace stressors that diminishes when the workplace stressors are removed. Taking this perspective, strains are part of the concurrent response to stressors and continuously fluctuate over time along with stressor levels (Garst et al., 2000).

There are theoretical reasons to expect that relations between synchronous chronic stressors and strains strengthen over time. The logic behind this prediction draws from conservation of resources theory (Hobfoll, 1989) and allostatic load theory (McEwen, 1998). According to conservation of resources theory, individuals strive to maintain and gain resources that help them respond to demands. Critical resources include time, energies, motivation, support and personal characteristics such as self-efficacy, with losses of or threats to these resources leading to stress. Workers must use resources to meet work demands, resulting in the cumulative depletion of those resources and causing strain (Schaufeli & Bakker, 2004). Conversely, the resources that workers have to cope with demands can reduce or "buffer" the effect of stressors on strains (de Jonge & Dormann, 2006). According to allostatic load theory (McEwen, 1998), bodily systems make physical accommodations to facilitate necessary responses to stressors and these accommodations use up resources. When stressors are prolonged, the accommodations, such as increased heart rate and blood pressure, become more permanent and constitute one's allostatic load. Thus, allostatic load increases over time even if one's stressor level does not change, as long as one's exposure is chronic (Ganzel, Morris, & Wethington, 2010), resulting in the cumulative depletion of one's physical, and presumably psychological, resources over time. This cumulative resource depletion is similar to what would be expected according to conservation of resources theory.

Taking the view proposed by these two theories, workers exposed to chronic stressors may experience a cumulative net loss of resources that gradually decreases their ability to effectively cope with the demands of work and increases the effects of chronic stressors across time. Frese and Zapf (1988) describe this type of change in effects as an *accumulation* model. For example, workers early in their tenure may replenish work-related energy loss during rest periods such that the effect of work stressors on fatigue and exhaustion is initially weak. However, if workers fail to completely replenish their energy and other resources over time, this may eventually increase the effect of stressors on strains as nonphysical resources become depleted and allostatic physical accommodations are made. Workers in demanding situations have been shown to have more difficulty detaching from work during nonwork hours (Sonnentag, Binnewies, & Mojza, 2010), and this failure to psychologically detach is associated with poor sleep quality (Sonnentag, Binnewies, & Mojza, 2008). Chronic work demands have also been found to be associated with higher baseline arousal levels that can in turn result in adrenal degeneration and weakening over time (Dienstbier, 1989; Schaubroeck & Ganster, 1993). Unpleasant psychological states, which may result from stressors, are known to reduce self-efficacy (Seo & Ilies, 2009) and this could also decrease one's capacity to cope with future stressors, creating a resource loss spiral (Demerouti, Bakker, & Bulters, 2004), and leading to less adaptive coping (Holahan & Moos, 1991). These perspectives all point to a potential increase in synchronous strain reactions to stressors over time.

Research Question 1: Do synchronous chronic occupational stressor-strain effects increase over time?

Lagged effects of stressors on strains

In addition to their synchronous effects cited above, chronic stressors may have longer-term physical and mental effects that take time to develop (Ganzel et al., 2010). Such effects, which have an incubation period, have been labelled *lagged* or *sleeper* effects (Garst et al., 2000). Quantitatively, lagged effects refer to the extent to which stressors at one point in time predict strains at a later point in time, controlling for strains at the initial point in time (i.e. controlling for the synchronous reactions). Such effects can also be operationalized as the extent to which stressor levels predict the trajectory, or slope, of strains over time.

Much of the logic predicting the existence of lagged effects is similar to the rationale predicting increases in synchronous short-term reactions to chronic stressors discussed above. As suggested in conservation of resources theory (Hobfoll, 1989) and allostatic load theory (McEwen, 1998), workers use up resources and make allostatic accommodations when responding to stressors. This depletion and accommodation in turn may increase strain in the future beyond any short-term immediate increases in strain by reducing one's resources to cope with future stressors. Such lagged effects are expected to take time to form. As noted above, allostatic load is a function of the cumulative exposure to stressors, not just current exposure, and cumulative exposure by definition increases over time.

Although there is a theoretical basis for lagged chronic stressor effects, empirical research to this point has failed to reach firm conclusions about how large these effects tend to be, how consistent they are across studies, and how they change across time. Dormann and Zapf (2002) suggested that a time period of at least two years is needed for lagged effects of chronic workplace stressors to emerge. Other researchers have found evidence suggesting that time lags of one year are long enough to see lagged chronic stressor effects peak (de Lange, Taris, Kompier, Houtman, & Bongers, 2004). As time passes the stressors of the workers are also likely to change, eventually diminishing the influence of the stressors that they were initially exposed to and that were measured at that time. This means that lagged effects would be expected to peak at some point and then decline. In this study, we meta-analytically assess these lagged effects across time to determine when they tend to peak.

Research Question 2: How large are lagged effects of occupational stressors on strains?

Research Question 3: How do lagged effects of chronic stressors on strains change over time?

Reverse causation effects

Reverse causation effects of strains on stressors have also received some attention in the work stress literature (e.g. de Lange et al., 2003). Reverse causation effects occur when high strain levels contribute to increases in stressors over time. The theoretical case for reverse causation effects is based on the notion that individuals experiencing strain, because of their diminished abilities and performance, end up in less desirable jobs with higher levels of stressors or at least come to perceive their jobs as more stressful. The effect of strain on future working conditions has been labelled by some as the "drift" hypothesis (Frese, 1982). Empirical research has shown that psychological and physical health are associated with cognitive performance (e.g. Austin, Mitchell, & Goodwin, 2001; Diestel, Cosmar, & Schmidt, 2013), self-efficacy and motivation (Mitchell, Hopper, Daniels, Georg-Falvy, & James, 1994) and general productivity (Ford, Cerasoli, Higgins, & DeCesare, 2011), providing some support for the rationale behind the drift hypothesis. Strained workers may also experience more negative feedback from their work environments given their impaired performance, increasing stressor levels. Furthermore, because workers in poorer psychological or physical health tend to have lower self-efficacy (e.g. Mitchell et al., 1994), they may appraise future demands as more challenging or threatening, even if those demands do not change. The evaluation, or appraisal, of a potential occupational stressor as benign, challenging or threatening, is integral to the stress response process (Lazarus & Folkman, 1984) and these appraisals may change over time. Thus, workers in poorer psychological health may come to appraise the same working conditions as more challenging or demanding, resulting in a reverse causation effect of strains on subsequent perceived stressors.

As with lagged effects, it is not clear how long reverse causation effects take to develop and how they change over time. Recent work by Judge and Hurst (2008) suggests that individuals who have positive core self-evaluations, one aspect of psychological health, early in their careers tend to experience more subsequent increases in pay and occupational status than those with less positive core self-evaluations. Such results indicate that workers with poor psychological health end up in less positive career trajectories. The adverse selection of strained workers into less desirable jobs may also result in impaired performance and well-being, in turn leading to fewer desirable employment options. Still, it is unclear how long these developments take, how large and consistent these effects are, and whether they eventually tend to diminish. Thus, we present the following research question.

Research Question 4: How large are reverse causation effects of strains on chronic occupational stressors and how do reverse causation effects of strains on chronic occupational stressors vary across time?

Differences across types of strain

There are some differences between low- and high-arousal strains that may result in differing synchronous and lagged effects. Using Russell's (1980) affective circumplex as a framework, high-arousal strains are those that involve high levels of activation and include anxiety and irritation, whereas low-arousal strains are those that involve low levels of activation and include depression, exhaustion and fatigue. Increases in arousal and activation are part of the immediate stress response to demanding or threatening situations (Gendolla & Krusken, 2002; Wright, Shaw, & Jones, 1990). High-arousal states help individuals mobilize the energy needed to respond to demands. Spector and Jex's (1998) review of their Quantitative Workload Inventory found stronger cross-sectional correlations between workload and anxiety than between workload and depression, suggesting that high-arousal states such as anxiety are more strongly associated with concurrent stressors.

The stronger synchronous associations between occupational stressors and high-arousal strains than between stressors and low-arousal strains point to two competing expectations. First, if short-term high-arousal reactions are stronger, this may result in weaker lagged effects on high-arousal strains because most of the effect occurs relatively immediately, leaving less room for a delayed effect. Alternatively, individuals who become chronically exposed to stressors may develop chronically high baseline arousal in anticipation of future stressors (Ganzel et al., 2010); this may occur to a greater degree with high-arousal than low-arousal strains, as low-arousal strains are not as functional in adapting to chronic demands. Hence, stronger synchronous effects of chronic stressors on high-arousal strains may also lead to stronger lagged effects on high-arousal strains. Therefore, we pose the following research question.

Research question 5: Are there differences in lagged effects across low- and high-arousal strains?

Method

This study's questions were addressed via a meta-analysis of relevant longitudinal panel studies. This involved a literature search, coding and calculation of synchronous, lagged and reverse causation effect sizes across studies.

Search procedures

Three different search procedures were used to obtain published literature reporting multi-wave panel studies where chronic occupational stressors and strains were measured at more than one point in time so that synchronous effects, and either lagged or reverse causation effects (or both), could be computed. First, we retrieved all articles referenced in three thorough narrative reviews of longitudinal stress research (de Lange et al., 2003; Sonnentag & Frese, 2003; Zapf, Dormann, & Frese, 1996). Second, we conducted keyword searches using the PsycInfo database. To identify articles reporting stressor-strain effects we used the following keywords in the search: *longitudinal*, *occupational*, *employee*, *organizational*, *stress*, *strain*, *stressor* and *health*. We searched for articles that combined "longitudinal" as a keyword with any of the other keywords. These searches yielded 79, 17, 85, 201, 20, 3 and 398 matches for searches with "longitudinal" plus each of the seven keywords, respectively. Third, manual searches were conducted of the following journals: *Journal of Applied Psychology*, *Academy of Management Journal*, *Journal of Organizational Behavior*, *Journal of Occupational Health Psychology*, *Journal of Vocational Behavior*, *Work & Stress*, *Organizational Behavior and Human Decision Processes*, *Journal of Management*, *Personnel Psychology* and *International Journal of Stress Management*. These 10 journals were selected for the manual search because of their rigorous publication standards and the frequency with which they publish occupational stress research. We selected 1975 as the starting point for our manual search given that prior to 1975 occupational stress research was not commonly published in organizational research journals. The manual searches were conducted by two trained undergraduate students and the first and second authors.

Additional search procedures were used to obtain unpublished literature that reported information relevant to our analyses. First, we searched the ProQuest Dissertations & Theses database for all articles with *stress* and *longitudinal* in the abstract, title, keyword or subject heading (that is, in all search fields except the man text). This search resulted in 2301 hits, the vast majority of which were not business or psychology dissertations due to the inclusiveness of the ProQuest database. This search also yielded many dissertations that were not retrievable given that the search spanned the entire twentieth century. Still, after a review of all abstracts from this search and attempts to gain access to the dissertations, several dissertations were retrieved, five of which were ultimately found to report information on lagged effects that had not been reported in a subsequent journal article. In addition, we contacted authors of conference presentations from the 2007–2011 Society for Industrial-Organizational Psychology conferences that appeared to report information that would be relevant to this analysis. We also sent a request out to an occupational health psychology LISTSERV requesting unpublished data. Usable unpublished data from two samples were obtained.

Coding and calculations for stressor-strain effects

Regarding chronic stressors, we included articles that measured social stressors, task stressors, demands or workload, role stressors or general unspecified stressors. Regarding strains, we included articles measuring exhaustion (including emotional exhaustion), fatigue, physical symptoms, depression, irritation, anxiety or general psychological ill-health/distress. A study was included if it reported enough information to (1) compute a lagged effect of a stressor on a strain or, (2) compute a reverse causation effect of a strain on a stressor (see the next paragraph for more detail). In all, 68 independent samples met this criterion. A reference list of all studies can be obtained by contacting the first author.

To assess synchronous, lagged and reverse causation effects, up to six correlations were recorded for each pair of time points in each study where stressors and strains were measured: the cross-sectional (or synchronous) correlation between the stressor and the strain at Time 1, the cross-sectional correlation between the stressor and the strain at Time 2, the correlation between the stressor at Time 1 and the strain at Time 2, the correlation between the strain at Time 1 and the stressor at Time 2, the correlation between the strain at Time 1 and the same strain at Time 2, and the correlation between the stressor at Time 1 and the same stressor at Time 2. By recording each of these correlations, we were able to (1) assess change in the stressor-strain correlation across time while accounting for the chronicity of the stressor (i.e. the correlation between Time 1 and Time 2 stressors), (2) compute beta weight coefficients for the stressor at Time 1, controlling for baseline strain, in the prediction of strain at Time 2 (i.e. lagged effects), and (3) compute beta weights for the strain at Time 1, controlling for baseline stressors, in the prediction of the stressor at Time 2 (i.e. reverse causation effects). A study was only included in this meta-analysis if enough information was reported to make these computations. For studies with more than two waves of data, all possible waves were recorded. For example, a panel study with three waves would have three sets of correlations, those for Time 1 and Time 2, those for Time 1 and Time 3 and those for Time 2 and Time 3.

The first author coded information from all studies. A random subset of 12 articles (17.4%) was also coded by one of the co-authors. For the data elements used in the study, inter-rater agreement was near perfect. All points of disagreement involved coding a different sample size based on missing data, with the sample size differences too small to have a substantive influence on the results. Because none of the differences had a substantive effect on the analysis we determined that the first author's coding was sufficiently accurate to draw conclusions from the rest of the data.

For the computation of lagged and reverse causation effects, the formula given in Cohen, Cohen, West, and Aiken (2003, p. 68) was used to compute the beta weight for the predictor in a regression equation including the predictor at Time 1 and the outcome at Time 1 as predictors of the outcome at Time 2. This method is consistent with Zapf et al.'s (1996) guidelines. These computations were performed for each individual lagged or reverse causation effect. For each effect, we computed two lagged effects. One effect was computed using correlations that were corrected for unreliability *prior* to entry into the formula. Thus, the corrected lagged effects were based on correlations that were first corrected for unreliability and then entered into the above formula. When the original study did not report the reliability of a stressor or a strain, the mean reliability, .82 or .85 for stressor or strain, respectively, was imputed and used to compute the corrected correlation. Physical symptoms scales are causal indicator scales, meaning that they are composed of conceptually distinct components (i.e. distinct symptoms) that do not necessarily reflect the same underlying construct. When this is the case, measures of internal consistency are not relevant. Thus, the reliability for measures of physical symptoms was considered to be 1 (Spector & Jex, 1998). We also computed lagged effects based on correlations that were *not* corrected for unreliability. Each subsequent analysis was conducted for both corrected and uncorrected lagged effects.

Analytical approach

In meta-analyzing the effects, Hunter and Schmidt's (2004) bare bones meta-analytic procedures were used. In computing the effects, when more than one synchronous, lagged or reverse causation effect for the *same* time point or time lag was reported in a single study, such as if multiple stressors were reported as having separate correlations with strains during the same time period, separate synchronous and lagged effects were first computed for each stressor-strain relation. Then the mean effects were computed and used to represent the effect for that study during that particular time point or time lag to avoid overweighting particular observations.

To test for changes in the *synchronous* stressor-strain effects across time, we analyzed models predicting the Time 2 stressor-strain correlation. The Time 1 stressor-strain correlation, the time lag length and the chronicity of the stressor (operationalized as the correlation between the stressor at Time 1 and the stressor at Time 2) were entered as predictors of the Time 2 stressor-strain correlation. We examined the chronicity of the stressors because stressor exposure would be expected to accumulate when stressors are chronic. Thus, the chronicity of the stressor should be accounted for. We then entered the interaction term for chronicity and time lag length to determine if the change in the synchronous stressor-strain correlation was dependent on the chronicity of the stressor. Because some studies included more than one effect (e.g. studies with more than two waves), the effect sizes were not all independent. Multilevel modelling through *HLM 6.06* (Raudenbush, Bryk, & Congdon, 2008) was used to account for this non-independence, with the sample treated as the Level-2 cluster variable. These analyses were also weighted by the sample size of the study (Steel & Kammeyer-Mueller, 2002).

To analyze changes in lagged and reverse causation effects across time, we used the same multilevel modelling approach as in the analysis of change in synchronous effects. For these analyses, the time lag, converted to years to ease the interpretation of the weights, was entered as a predictor of the lagged or reverse causation effect, followed by square and cubic terms to test for curvilinear relations between length of time lag and lagged or reverse causation effect size.

Results

Change in synchronous effects across time

The first research question asked whether and how synchronous stressor-strain effects (that is, those in which the strain changes concurrently with the stressor and both are measured at all time points) change across time. We meta-analyzed the synchronous correlations at Time 1 and at Time 2 for all instances where the stressor-strain correlation was measured at two points in time. If data at more than two time points were collected in a study, all pairs of time points were included in this analysis. These results are shown in Table 1. As seen in Table 1, the corrected and uncorrected synchronous correlations were not significantly different between Time 1 and Time 2 for any of the effects.

We then examined whether the synchronous effects tended to increase over longer time lags. The main effects of time lag and stressor chronicity (i.e. its stability – the degree to which the stressor level at Time 1 was correlated with the stressor level at Time 2) on change in the stressor-psychological strain correlation were not significant, $\gamma = -.005$ and $.009$, respectively for values corrected for unreliability, and $\gamma = -.005$ and $-.014$, respectively, for uncorrected values, all *n.s.* However, there was a significant interaction between stressor chronicity and time lag, $\gamma = .058$ for corrected values and $.067$ for uncorrected values, $p < .05$ for both. This meant that the synchronous stressor-strain effect tended to increase more over time for stressors that were relatively stable (i.e. chronic), than for stressors that were not. Figure 1 shows the best fit regression lines, which demonstrate this effect.

The same analysis was conducted for physical strain. Results showed a main effect for time lag, $\gamma = .024$ and $.020$ for corrected and uncorrected values, $p < .05$, and a marginally significant effect for chronicity using corrected values, $\gamma = .229$, $p = .052$. These results suggest that the synchronous stressor-physical strain correlations tended to increase over time. The interaction term between time lag and chronicity (i.e. degree of stability) was not significant, $\gamma = .001$ and $.013$ for corrected and uncorrected values, indicating that the increase in the stressor-physical strain correlation did not depend on the stability of the stressor over time. Overall, these results suggest that longer time lags were associated with larger increases in synchronous stressor-strain correlations. These increases were stronger for psychological strain when the stressors were high in chronicity (i.e. stable).

Lagged effects of stressors on strains

The bottom half of Table 1 shows the meta-analytic results for all lagged effects of stressors on strains (that is, effects of Time 1 stressors on Time 2 strain, controlling for Time 1 strain). The sample size-weighted mean lagged effect size for psychological strain

Table 1. Bare-bones meta-analytic cross-sectional, lagged main and reverse causation effects for psychological and physical strains.

	k	N	Mean effect based on corrected values	Mean effect based on uncorrected values	Var (r) corrected values	Var (r) uncorrected values	95% CI corrected values	95% CI uncorrected values
Psychological strain, synchronous effects								
Time 1	91	24,844	.351	.290	.015	.012	.340, .362	.279, .302
Time 2	91	24,844	.370	.308	.017	.013	.359, .381	.297, .319
Physical strain, synchronous effects								
Time 1	29	15,678	.121	.107	.006	.005	.105, .136	.092, .123
Time 2	29	15,678	.142	.129	.006	.005	.127, .158	.113, .144
Main lagged effects								
Psychological Strain	109	43,075	.030	.052	.003	.002	.021, .040	.043, .062
Physical Strain	38	19,550	.047	.043	.003	.002	.033, .061	.029, .057
Reverse causation effects								
Psychological Strain	91	27,304	.014	.061	.005	.003	.002, .026	.050, .073
Physical Strain	29	15,678	.036	.046	.002	.001	.020, .052	.031, .062

Note: k = number of effects from which values were calculated; N = total sample size; 95% CI = 95% confidence interval around weighted mean; Var (r) = variance in the observed values. Synchronous effects reported only for studies that report synchronous effects at Time 1 *and* Time 2.

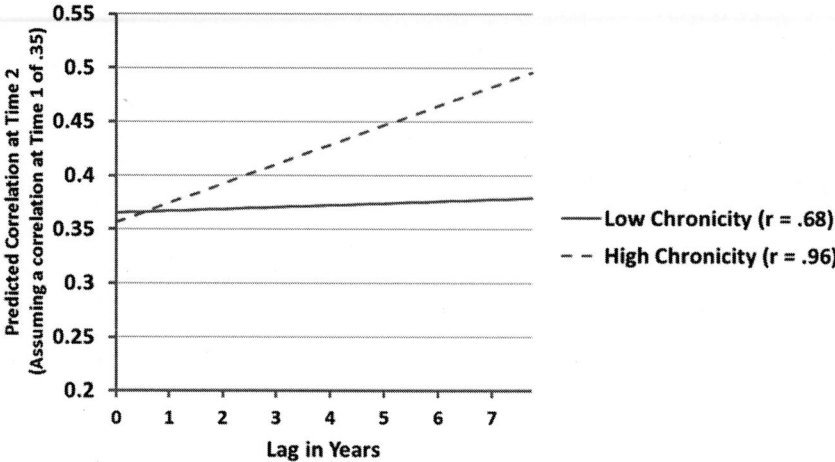

Figure 1.   Best fit regression lines showing changes in cross-sectional correlations between stressor and psychological strain across time and stressor chronicity. Chronicity represents the correlation between stressors at Time 1 and Time 2. Levels of chronicity represent 1 standard deviation above and below the mean chronicity of stressors (.82).

was .030 for corrected values and .052 for uncorrected values. We then examined models testing the effects of time lags on lagged effect sizes. In this examination, the time lag (in years) was first entered, followed by its square and cubic terms. The results (see Table 2) indicate no linear effect for the time lag based on corrected values and a negative effect based on uncorrected values, $\gamma = -.004$, $p < .05$. The coefficient for the square term was significant for corrected values, $\gamma = -.002$, $p < .05$, but not for uncorrected values. Finally, the cubic term was significant for the corrected values, $\gamma = .0004$, $p < .05$, and marginally significant for the uncorrected values, $\gamma = .0003$, $p < .10$. These results generally suggest that the lagged effects increased across time, then decreased, and eventually levelled out. As seen in Figure 2, which includes a plot of all lagged effects by time lag, there was wide variability in the lagged effects, although some of the deviant effects were based on small samples and carried comparatively less weight in the analysis. Based on the square and cubic trend lines, lagged effects peaked at about three years before decreasing to an asymptotic pattern after a lag of about seven years.

For physical strain, the sample-size weighted mean effects were .047 and .043 for corrected and uncorrected values (see Table 1). Results for models testing the effect of time lag length (see Table 2) found no effects of time lag on the lagged effect. Thus, there was no discernible pattern in how lagged effects on physical strain varied across time.

Reverse causation effects

Reverse causation effects, operationalized as the beta weight for Time 1 strain predicting Time 2 stressors, controlling for Time 1 stressors in the same regression model, were analyzed using the same method as for the lagged effects. As reported in Table 1, the reverse causation effects of psychological strain on chronic stressors were .014 and .061 for corrected and uncorrected values, respectively. The lower effects for corrected values were probably due to the fact that the Time 1-Time 2 stressor correlation often

Table 2. Weighted multilevel models predicting main and reverse causation lagged effects with time lag length (in years).

	Coefficient (γ) using corrected values	Coefficient (γ) using uncorrected values	Coefficient (γ) using corrected values	Coefficient (γ) using uncorrected values	Coefficient (γ) using corrected values	Coefficient (γ) using uncorrected values	Coefficient (γ) using corrected values	Coefficient (γ) using uncorrected values
	Psychological Strain (109 effects)		Physical Strain (38 effects)		Psychological Strain reverse causation (91 effects)		Physical Strain reverse causation (29 effects)	
Step 1								
Intercept (γ_{00})	.031*	.059*	.060*	.055*	−.004	.057*	.010	.029*
Years (γ_{10})	−.001	−.004*	−.004	−.004	.009*	.004*	.011*	.008*
Step 2								
Intercept (γ_{00})	.016*	.051*	.064*	.056*	−.007	.058*	.001	.028^
Years (γ_{10})	.016*	.004	−.008	−.005	.013^	.003	.023*	.009
Years² (γ_{20})	−.002*	−.001	−.001	.000	−.001	.000	−.002	.000
Step 3								
Intercept (γ_{00})	.000	.040*	.030	.024	−.011	.057*	.002	.033
Years (γ_{10})	.041*	.021^	.039	.040	.020	.003	.018	.001
Years² (γ_{20})	−.008*	−.005^	−.015	−.014	−.002	.000	.000	.003
Years³ (γ_{30})	.0004*	.0003^	.001	.001^	.000	.000	.000	.000

Note: Coefficients are unstandardized. Intercepts were allowed to vary randomly across studies. *p < .05. ^p < .10. ²squared term. ³cubic term. Models were weighted by study sample size when estimated.

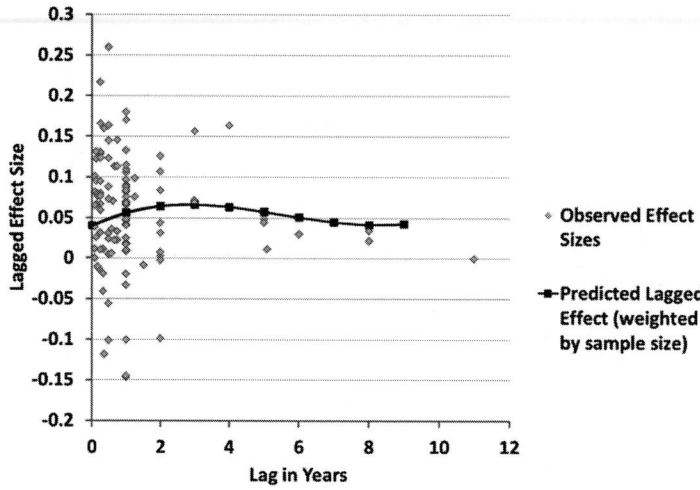

Figure 2. Plot of lagged effects on psychological strain, by time lag, for the studies analyzed. Note: The curvilinear trend lines illustrate the predicted lagged effect size across time lags based on weighted multilevel modelling.

approached or reached 1 after correction for reliability, leaving very little or no additional variance to explain. We examined the effect of time lag on the size of the reverse causation effects (see Table 2) and found that the linear term for time lag was significant and positive, $\gamma = .009$ and $.004$ for corrected and uncorrected values, $p < .05$ for both, whereas the square and cubic terms were not significant. This suggests that the magnitude of reverse causation effects of psychological strain on stressors tended to increase across time without eventually decreasing (see Figure 3 for a plot of these effects). The mean reverse causation effects for physical strain were $.036$ and $.046$. Analyses revealed that the physical strain reverse causation effects also tended to increase over time, $\gamma = .011$ and $.008$ for corrected and uncorrected values, $p < .05$ for both. Thus, the effects of time lags on reverse causation effects were similar across psychological and physical strains.

Differences across strains

We separated the lagged effects according to strains to examine if there were differences across the types of strains. These results are shown in Table 3. We used non-overlapping confidence intervals as the criterion for significant differences across strains. The mean time lag was also computed for each cell for informational purposes as it is possible that the type of strain was confounded with time lag. Lagged effects on high-arousal strains (i.e. anxiety, irritation and tension), $\beta = .059$, were stronger than for exhaustion/fatigue, $\beta = .018$, when using corrected values. Reverse causation effects showed no significant differences across strains. Reverse causation effects of psychological well-being/overall distress, $\beta = .086$, were stronger than those for depression, $\beta = .041$, and anxiety/irritation, $\beta = .028$, using uncorrected values. No other significant differences across the strains were found.

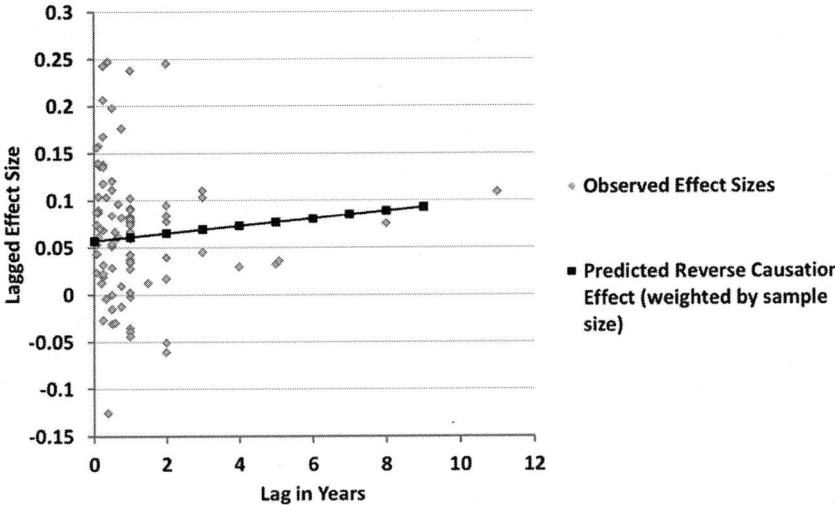

Figure 3. Plot of reverse causation effects of psychological strain on stressors, by time lag (in years).
Note: The linear trend line illustrates the predicted lagged effect size across time lags based on weighted multilevel modelling.

Discussion

The goals of this study were to examine variability in synchronous and lagged occupational stressor-strain effects across time, link this variability to theoretical perspectives on the role of time in occupational stress reactions, and advance the field's knowledge on the consistency of lagged effects across studies and the power needed to detect them. The results suggest that synchronous stressor-strain effects tend to strengthen over time, with stressor-psychological strain effects increasing especially when workers were consistently exposed to those stressors. The magnitude of lagged effects on psychological strain, which were modest in size, tended to increase for about three years before declining, whereas lagged effects on physical strain showed no clear pattern. In contrast, reverse causation effects of both psychological and physical strain on stressors tended to increase in a linear pattern over time. Finally, the results showed substantial variability in the lagged effects across studies. The lagged and reverse causation effect size means, which ranged from .043 to .061, suggest that large sample sizes are needed to detect lagged effects reliably. These results have important theoretical and methodological implications for occupational stress research.

Changes in synchronous stressor-strain effects across time

The theoretical perspectives presented in this study's Introduction suggest that prolonged exposure to stressors results in an increase in allostatic load and a net loss of resources. This cumulative loss decreases one's ability to cope with and respond to stressors in the future and results in stronger synchronous stress reactions over time. Empirical results from this analysis support this theoretical position, as cross-sectional correlations between stressors and strains tended to increase over time in longitudinal studies, with this increase becoming larger when there was a longer period of time between measurement occasions.

Table 3. Meta-analytic mean lagged and reverse causation effects across strains.

	k	Mean time lag (in months)	N	β (corrected values)	β (uncorrected values)	Var (r) corrected	Var (r) uncorrected	95% CI corrected	95% CI uncorrected
Lagged effects on psychological strain, by psychological strain									
Exhaustion/Fatigue	46	13.89	20,421	.018	.062	.0029	.0055	.004, .032	.048, .075
Anxiety/Irritation/Tension	20	20.55	5426	.059	.075	.0114	.0120	.033, .086	.048, .101
Depression	38	16.37	13,123	.036	.046	.0035	.0047	.019, .053	.029, .063
Psychological well-being/ Overall distress	43	12.02	20,836	.043	.052	.0035	.0051	.029, .057	.039, .066
Reverse causation effects, by strain									
Exhaustion/Fatigue	40	13.91	15,439	.007	.077	.0061	.0080	−.009, .022	.061, .092
Anxiety/Irritation/Tension	20	19.13	5102	.007	.028	.0085	.0064	−.019, .034	.001, .056
Depression	34	14.94	11,555	.021	.041	.0028	.0042	.003, .039	.023, .059
Psychological well-being/ Overall distress	32	9.41	5902	.030	.086	.0101	.0119	.005, .056	.060, .111

Note: k = number of effects from which values were calculated; N = total sample size; β = weighted mean lagged effect; 95% CI = 95% confidence interval around weighted mean; Var (r) = variance in the observed effects.

Also interesting was that, for psychological strains, chronic or consistent stressors, as operationalized by the stressor autocorrelations, resulted in greater increases in synchronous stressor-strain effects. This further supports the view that prolonged exposure to the same stressors tends to increase synchronous stress reactions. These findings are also consistent with a dose-response effect of chronic stressors such that cumulative exposure, not just current exposure, determines one's level of strain. This type of effect has also been found elsewhere (Chandola, Brunner, & Marmot, 2006).

Changes in lagged and reverse causation effects across time

Lagged effects of stressors on psychological and physical strains were significant but relatively weak by conventional effect size standards. Considering lagged effects are often used as more rigorous tests of causality than cross-sectional, synchronous effects, it is important to note that lagged effects are theoretically different from synchronous effects and are smaller and more difficult to detect. There was also considerable variability in lagged effects, some of which could be explained by the time lag. Lagged effects on psychological strain tended to increase up to a period of about three years before declining. As noted in the introduction, some effects of occupational stressors on strain, through the cumulative depletion of one's resources and increases in allostatic load, are expected to occur after some time has elapsed, and these results confirm this view.

Although small by conventional standards, the lagged effects were statistically significant for large samples and effects of this size can still be compelling, particularly when considering dependent variables like strain that are fairly resistant to change (Prentice & Miller, 1992). Dispositions during adulthood, which underlie a significant portion of negative psychological strains, tend to be relatively stable (Roberts, Caspi, & Moffitt, 2001; Watson & Walker, 1996). Given the limited proportion of variance in psychological and physical strain that tends to change over time, the fact that some of the change is attributable to occupational stressors is notable. This suggests that some of the effects of job stressors on occupational strain have a delayed onset and that work stressors explain some of the changes we find in adult psychological and physical well-being over time. It is also worth noting that even relatively small effect sizes in predicting health can result in nontrivial increases in risk for those in the most risky or stressful situations. An effect size of .06 converts to an odds ratio of 1.24 using recommended formulas (Haddock, Rindskopf, & Shadish, 1998; Hasselblad & Hedges, 1995). This would suggest that workers in high-stressor jobs are at a 24% greater risk for developing increased psychological strain in the future than those in low-stressor jobs. Such effects, despite their size, would have consequences for a large number of workers.

Reverse causation effects of psychological and physical strain on chronic stressors were also relatively weak. The mean corrected correlation between Time 1 and Time 2 stressors was .82, which means that chronic occupational stressors tend to be stable for most people. To the extent that chronic stressors changed, physical and psychological strain explained a significant proportion of this change. The reverse causation effects of psychological strain were also larger for longer time lags, suggesting that reverse causation effects increase with time. Perhaps changes in chronic stressors through the aforementioned drift hypothesis (Frese, 1982) take a longer time to occur than lagged effects of stressors on strains but are also more difficult to reverse. These results are consistent with Judge and Hurst's (2008) finding that poor psychological well-being predicts a less positive career trajectory.

Methodological implications

One methodological issue that emerged from our results was that large samples are needed to ensure adequate power to detect lagged and reverse causation effects in individual studies. At any given point in time, most employees in most occupational stress studies have already experienced to some degree the chronic stressors that are being measured and thus have already developed reactions to those stressors. It is not surprising then that the size of lagged effects among job incumbents tends to be small. To have a power of .80 to detect a correlation of .10, larger than the mean lagged effect size found here, a sample size of 783 would be required (Cohen et al., 2003, p. 654). Because of the size of these expected effects, large sample sizes are needed for powerful tests of hypotheses about change in strain in observational studies. Effect sizes of this magnitude are not necessarily trivial, considering the arguments made above; they just require large samples sizes to detect with confidence.

These results also suggest that researchers should consider measuring occupational histories to account for past exposures to stressors that may have implications for synchronous and lagged effects. Little research to date on chronic work stressors has incorporated and tested theories about the effects of past exposure on occupational strain. However, composition models combining current and past stressor exposures may be useful in improving understanding and prediction of strain.

These results and our accompanying theoretical review suggest that both synchronous and lagged effects are important and deserve research attention. However, they reflect theoretically different causal phenomena and have very different effects sizes and sample size requirements. If a researcher is substantively interested in psychological or physical strains that have a delayed onset after exposure to occupational stressors, then lagged effects may be more appropriate, but a large sample will likely be needed to reliably detect these effects. However, if the effects of stressors on strains are not expected to have a delayed onset, synchronous effects may be more appropriate, with the caveat that there could be greater ambiguity when interpreting the causal directions among the stressors and strains.

Practical implications

The changes in synchronous stressor-strain relations as a function of the chronicity (i.e. the stability) of stressors have practical implications for organizations attempting to manage employee stress. This study suggests that when chronic stressor levels are maintained, workers' synchronous stress reactions increase substantially over time. In contrast, when these occupational stressor levels are less stable, the synchronous reactions do not appear to increase as much. Although it is ideal to minimize chronic stressors at work when possible, if it is impossible to eliminate occupational stressors entirely, then giving workers extended breaks from demands may allow them to replenish their resources and reduce strains over time. It is known from past research that acute (e.g. nightly) breaks from chronic work demands have benefits (Sonnentag et al., 2008). More extended reductions in demands may also give workers a chance to replenish their resources and reduce their cumulative load. Further research is needed on the effectiveness of strategies such as these, but the results and theoretical reasoning presented here suggest that allowing for breaks from occupational stressors, and thereby reducing the cumulative demands on workers, may attenuate the effect of chronic occupational stressors on employee strain.

Limitations

One primary limitation of note in this study is in the interpretation of the synchronous stressor-strain effects that we analyzed. Our conclusions on the synchronous stressor-strain effects must take into account the difficulty in determining causal direction from cross-sectional correlations. Theory and laboratory research would suggest that stressors do indeed play a causal role in strains, but it is impossible to empirically rule out reverse causality in cross-sectional field observations. However, logic dictates that synchronous stressor-strain effects occur concurrently and therefore are most evident in cross-sectional effects, even though these cross-sectional effects may also reflect some reverse causation or spurious effects. Thus, the limitations of cross-sectional research must be considered when interpreting results from synchronous stressor-strain effects.

A second limitation of our analysis is the potential for a "file-drawer" publication bias. It is possible that studies that are published are more likely to have significant lagged effects than studies that remain unpublished. Because this analysis included mostly published studies, these results may overstate the true size of lagged effects. Still, it is also worth noting that many of the lagged effects recorded for this analysis were not the central point of the studies they were drawn from. Thus, the lagged effects were not always critical in the publication of these studies, meaning they may be less likely to be systematically biased upward. This feature does not eliminate publication bias but may have reduced its magnitude here.

Conclusion

The results of this review and meta-analysis of longitudinal studies provide new insights into the role of time in synchronous, lagged and reverse causation effects among chronic occupational stressors and strains. Findings from the analyses suggest that occupational stressors become more strongly related to strains over time. Furthermore, analyses of lagged effects suggest that chronic occupational stressors on average predict modest increases in strain, with these effects peaking after about three years and tending to be slightly stronger for high-arousal than for low-arousal strains. Reverse causation effects of psychological strain were similarly modest and tended to increase over time.

These findings are generally consistent with conservation of resources and allostatic load theories, suggesting that cumulative exposure to chronic work stressors increases reactions to those stressors. Still, there was much unexplained variability in lagged and reverse causation effects across studies, indicating that other factors may help explain how chronic stressor-strain effects change over time. Therefore, there remains a need for further research on the development of synchronous and lagged stressor-strain relations across time and methods for organizations and individuals to prevent the negative outcomes of chronic occupational stressors.

References

N.B. A reference list of all studies used in the analyses can be obtained by contacting the first author.

Austin, M., Mitchell, P., & Goodwin, G. M. (2001). Cognitive deficits in depression: Possible implications for functional neuropathology. *British Journal of Psychiatry 178*, 200–206.

Bono, J. E., & McNamara, G. (2011). Publishing in AMJ- part 2: Research design. *Academy of Management Journal, 54*, 657–660.

Chandola, T., Brunner, E., & Marmot, M. (2006). Chronic stress at work and the metabolic syndrome: Prospective study. *British Medical Journal 332*, 521–525.

Cohen, J., Cohen, P., West, S. G., & Aiken, L. S. (2003). *Applied multiple regression/correlation analysis for the behavioral sciences*. Mahwah, NJ: Lawrence Erlbaum.

de Jonge, J., & Dormann, C. (2006). Stressors, resources, and strain at work: A longitudinal test of the triple-match principle. *Journal of Applied Psychology, 91*, 1359–1374.

de Lange, A. H., Taris, T. W., Kompier, M. A. J., Houtman, I. L. D., & Bongers, P. M. (2003). "The *very* best of the millennium": Longitudinal research and the demand-control-(*support*) model. *Journal of Occupational Health Psychology, 8*, 282–305.

de Lange, A. H., Taris, T. W., Kompier, M. A. J., Houtman, I. L. D., & Bongers, P. M. (2004). The relationships between work characteristics and mental health: Examining normal, reversed, and reciprocal relationships in a 4-wave study. *Work & Stress, 18*, 149–166.

Demerouti, E., Bakker, A. B., & Bulters, A. J. (2004). The loss spiral of work pressure, work-home interference and exhaustion: Reciprocal relations in a three-wave study. *Journal of Vocational Behavior, 64*(1), 131–149.

Dienstbier, R. A. (1989). Arousal and physiological toughness: Implications for mental and physical health. *Psychological Review, 96*(1), 84–100.

Diestel, S., Cosmar, M., & Schmidt, K. H. (2013). Burnout and impaired cognitive functioning: The role of executive control in the performance of cognitive tasks. *Work & Stress, 27*, 164–180.

Dormann, C., & Zapf, D. (2002). Social stressors at work, irritation, and depressive symptoms: Accounting for unmeasured third variables in a multi-wave study. *Journal of Occupational and Organizational Psychology, 75*(1), 33–58.

Ford, M. T., Cerasoli, C. P., Higgins, J. A., & DeCesare, A. L. (2011). Relationships between psychological, physical, and behavioural health and work performance: A review and meta-analysis. *Work & Stress, 25*, 185–204.

Frese, M. (1982). Occupational socialization and psychological development: An underemphasized research perspective in industrial psychology. *Journal of Occupational Psychology, 55*, 209–224.

Frese, M. (1999). Social support as a moderator of the relationship between work stressors and psychological dysfunctioning: A longitudinal study with objective measures. *Journal of Occupational Health Psychology, 4*, 179–192.

Frese, M., & Zapf, D. (1988). Methodological issues in the study of work stress: Objective vs. subjective measurement of work stress and the question of longitudinal studies. In C. L. Cooper & R. Payne (Eds.), *Causes, coping, and consequents of stress at work* (pp. 375–411). Chichester: Wiley.

Ganzel, B. L., Morris, P. A., & Wethington, E. (2010). Allostasis and the human brain: Integrating models of stress from the social and life sciences. *Psychological Review, 117*, 134–174.

Garst, H., Frese, M., & Molenaar, P. C. M. (2000). The temporal factor of change in stressor-strain relationships: A growth curve model on a longitudinal study in East Germany. *Journal of Applied Psychology, 85*, 417–438.

Gendolla, G. H. E., & Krusken, J. (2002). The joint effect of informational mood impact and performance-contingent consequences on effort-related cardiovascular response. *Journal of Personality and Social Psychology, 83*, 271–283.

Haddock, C., Rindskopf, D., & Shadish, W. R. (1998). Using odds ratios as effect sizes for meta-analysis of dichotomous data: A primer on methods and issues. *Psychological Methods, 3*, 339–353.

Hasselblad, V., & Hedges, L. V. (1995). Meta-analysis of screening and diagnostic tests. *Psychological Bulletin, 117*, 167–178.

Hobfoll, S. E. (1989). Conservation of resources: A new attempt at conceptualizing stress. *American Psychologist, 44*, 513–524.

Holahan, C. J., & Moos, R. H. (1991). Life stressors, personal and social resources, and depression: A 4-year structural model. *Journal of Abnormal Psychology*, *100*(1), 31–38.

Hunter, J. E., & Schmidt, F. L. (2004). *Methods of meta-analysis: Correcting error and bias in research findings* (2nd ed.). Thousand Oaks, CA: Sage.

Judge, T. A., & Hurst, C. (2008). How the rich (and happy) get richer (and happier): Relationship of core self-evaluations to trajectories in attaining work success. *Journal of Applied Psychology*, *93*, 849–863.

Kahn, R. L., & Byosiere, P. (1992). Stress in organizations. In M. D. Dunnette & L. M. Hough (Eds.), *Handbook of industrial and organizational psychology* (2nd ed., Vol. 3, pp. 571–650). Palo Alto, CA: Consulting Psychologists Press.

Lazarus, R. S., & Folkman, S. (1984). *Stress, appraisal, and coping*. New York, NY: Springer.

Maslach, C., & Leiter, M. P. (2008). Early predictors of job burnout and engagement. *Journal of Applied Psychology*, *93*, 498–512.

McEwen, B. S. (1998). Stress, adaptation, and disease: Allostasis and allostatic load. *Annals of the New York Academy of Sciences*, *840*(1), 33–44.

Mitchell, T. R., Hopper, H., Daniels, D., George-Falvy, J., & James, L. R. (1994). Predicting self-efficacy and performance during skill acquisition. *Journal of Applied Psychology*, *79*, 506–517.

Mitchell, T. R., & James, L. R. (2001). Building better theory: Time and the specification of when things happen. *Academy of Management Review*, *26*, 530–547.

Nixon, A. E., Mazzola, J. J., Bauer, J., Krueger, J. R., & Spector, P. E. (2011). Can work make you sick? A meta-analysis of the relationships between job stressors and physical symptoms. *Work & Stress*, *25*, 1–22.

Prentice, D. A., & Miller, D. T. (1992). When small effects are impressive. *Psychological Bulletin*, *112*, 160–164.

Raudenbush, S., Bryk, A., & Congdon, R. (2008). HLM (6.06) [Computer software]. Lincolnwood, IL: Scientific Software International.

Roberts, B. W., Caspi, A., & Moffitt, T. E. (2001). The kids are alright: Growth and stability in personality development from adolescence to adulthood. *Journal of Personality and Social Psychology*, *81*, 670–683.

Russell, J. A. (1980). A circumplex model of affect. *Journal of Personality and Social Psychology*, *39*, 1161–1178.

Schaubroeck, J., & Ganster, D. C. (1993). Chronic demands and responsivity to challenge. *Journal of Applied Psychology*, *78*(1), 73–85.

Schaufeli, W. B., & Bakker, A. B. (2004). Job demands, job resources, and their relationship with burnout and engagement: A multi-sample study. *Journal of Organizational Behavior*, *25*, 293–315.

Schonfeld, I. S. (1996). Relation of negative affectivity to self-reports of job stressors and psychological outcomes. *Journal of Occupational Health Psychology*, *1*, 397–412.

Seo, M.-G., & Ilies, R. (2009). The role of self-efficacy, goal, and affect in dynamic motivational self-regulation. *Organizational Behavior and Human Decision Processes*, *109*(2), 120–133.

Sonnentag, S., Binnewies, C., & Mojza, E. J. (2008). "Did you have a nice evening?" A day level study on recovery experiences, sleep, and affect. *Journal of Applied Psychology*, *93*, 674–684.

Sonnentag, S., Binnewies, C., & Mojza, E. J. (2010). Staying well and engaged when demands are high: The role of psychological detachment. *Journal of Applied Psychology*, *95*, 965–976.

Sonnentag, S., & Frese, M. (2003). Stress in organizations. In W. C. Borman, D. R. Ilgen, & R. J. Klimoski (Eds.), *Handbook of psychology volume 12: Industrial and organizational psychology*. Hoboken, NJ: Wiley.

Spector, P. E., & Jex, S. M. (1998). Development of four self-report measures of job stressors and stain: Interpersonal conflict at work scale, organizational constraints scale, quantitative workload inventory, and physical symptoms inventory. *Journal of Occupational Health Psychology*, *3*, 356–367.

Steel, P. D., & Kammeyer-Mueller, J. D. (2002). Comparing meta-analytic moderator estimation techniques under realistic conditions. *Journal of Applied Psychology*, *87*(1), 96–111.

Watson, D., & Walker, L. M. (1996). The long-term stability and predictive validity of trait measures of affect. *Journal of Personality and Social Psychology*, *70*, 567–577.

Westman, M., & Eden, D. (1997). Effects of a respite from work on burnout: Vacation relief and fade-out. *Journal of Applied Psychology*, *82*, 516–527.

Wright, R. A., Shaw, L. L. & Jones, C. R. (1990). Task demand and cardiovascular response magnitude: Further evidence of the mediating role of success importance. *Journal of Personality and Social Psychology*, *59*, 1250–1260.

Zapf, D., Dormann, C., & Frese, M. (1996). Longitudinal studies in organizational stress research: A review of the literature with reference to methodological issues. *Journal of Occupational Health Psychology*, *1*, 145–169.

The effect of conflict at work on well-being: Depressive symptoms as a vulnerability factor

Laurenz L. Meier[a,b], Norbert K. Semmer[c] and Sven Gross[c]

[a]Department of Psychology, University of South Florida, Tampa, FL, USA; [b]Department of Psychology, University of Fribourg, Fribourg, Switzerland; [c]Department of Psychology, University of Bern, Bern, Switzerland

In occupational health research, aspects of psychological well-being, including depressive symptoms, have mainly been considered as an outcome. In this research, we examined the role of depressive symptoms as a moderator in the relationship between interpersonal conflict at work and psychological and physical well-being. We assumed that people with relatively high levels of chronic depressive symptoms react particularly strongly to conflict. We tested our hypotheses with a cross-sectional study ($N = 218$) and with a diary study over two weeks ($N = 127$). Both studies were conducted in Switzerland. The results of both studies showed that conflict was related to impaired psychological well-being (depressive mood and job satisfaction) and physical well-being (somatic complaints). In line with our assumption, this effect was particularly strong for people with high levels of chronic depressive symptoms. Thus, our findings suggest that conflict may lead to depressive symptoms, which make people even more vulnerable to conflicts, indicating a vicious circle with high psychological and economic costs.

Introduction

Previous research has clearly indicated that adverse work conditions are positively related to depressive symptoms (Bonde, 2008; Tennant, 2001). Prospective studies suggest that work stressors such as conflict are likely to increase depressive symptoms (e.g. Dormann & Zapf, 1999), but that depressive symptoms may also lead to an increase in experienced work stressors (e.g. Finne, Knardahl, & Lau, 2011). Thus, depressive symptoms can be considered both as a consequence and an antecedent of work stressors, pointing to a loss spiral. Hence, they may play a role in the pathogenesis of more severe psychological disorders such as major depression. However, depressive symptoms may be important beyond being a potential predictor and outcome. They may act as a moderator by aggravating the negative impact of work stressors on psychological and physical well-being, which would further strengthen the loss spiral. However, previous research has focused on depressive symptoms as outcome or predictor, but neglected its potential role as a moderator in the relationship between stressor and strain. In this paper, we present two studies that address this issue and help to extend our knowledge about the role of depressive symptoms in work stress. We focused on conflict as work stressor because conflict has been considered as particularly stressful (e.g. Bolger, DeLongis, Kessler, & Schilling, 1989) and because people with high levels of depressive symptoms are expected to be particularly vulnerable to such a social stressor.

Conflict at work and well-being

Interpersonal conflicts in the workplace may occur in diverse forms, ranging from minor disagreements between co-workers and supervisor to assaults on others, and they may be overt or covert (see Spector & Jex, 1998). Conflicts may refer to disagreements that are related to feelings of animosity (relationship conflict) or to disagreements regarding the best way to accomplish a task (task conflict) (e.g. Jehn, 1995). Conflicts are often associated with the experience of disrespect and interpersonal rejection; this is particularly true for relationship-related conflict (see De Dreu & Gelfand, 2008; Meier, Gross, Spector, & Semmer, 2013). Events involving interpersonal rejection are especially aversive because they undermine the fundamental need to belong to significant others and to maintain good interpersonal relationships (Baumeister & Leary, 1995).

Interpersonal conflict at work has been linked to various indicators of well-being, such as depressive symptoms, job satisfaction and somatic symptoms (e.g. Spector & Bruk-Lee, 2008). Most of this research is based on cross-sectional data. However, there are a few studies that examined associations between conflicts and well-being across time. With regard to rather long time lags (i.e. several months), Dormann and Zapf (1999) found that interpersonal conflict was prospectively related to depressive symptoms, at least when social support was low. With regard to very short time lags (i.e. hours), Ilies, Johnson, Judge, and Keeney (2011) and Meier et al. (2013) found that interpersonal conflict had short-term effects on negative mood. Thus, it is reasonable to assume that both chronic conflict and daily conflict episodes may impair well-being.

The moderating role of depressive symptoms

As mentioned above, depressive symptoms have been almost exclusively considered as an outcome variable, and research on conflict (Dormann & Zapf, 1999) and related stressors such as a bad team climate (Ylipaavalniemi et al., 2005) found lagged effects on depressive symptoms. In our research, however, we assumed not only that depressive symptoms are the result of conflicts, but also that people with depressive symptoms are more vulnerable to conflict (i.e. it strengthens the relationship between conflicts and well-being). In line with taxometric analyses showing that depressive symptoms are best conceptualized as a continuous construct (e.g. Prisciandaro & Roberts, 2005; Ruscio & Ruscio, 2000), we use the term depressive symptoms to denote a continuous variable (i.e. individual differences in depressive symptoms) rather than a clinical category such as major depressive disorder. The dimensional nature of depressive symptoms implies that clinically depressed individuals are to be found only in the high range of depressive symptoms (see Baldwin & Shean, 2006), and that people who are not clinically depressed (such as those in our sample) can still show quite some variance in depressive symptoms.

The theoretical rationale of an increased reactivity of people with a high level of depressive symptoms to conflicts is based on appraisal theory (Lazarus, 1991; Ellsworth & Scherer, 2003). According to this theory, people appraise (i) whether a situation threatens important needs and goals and hence is relevant for their well-being (primary appraisal) and (ii) whether efforts to cope with the situation might change the situation (secondary appraisal). Regarding primary appraisal, people with high levels of depressive symptoms have been found to be more dependent on others, having insecure feelings of belonging, fears of abandonment, and feelings of weakness and helplessness (Blatt, Quinlan, Chevron, McDonald, & Zuroff, 1982). Thus, negative situations that threaten the need to belong, such as conflicts (see above), are expected to be appraised as particularly threatening by people with relatively high depressive symptoms; in line with this, people with high levels of depressive symptoms react particularly strongly to interpersonal rejection (Nezlek, Kowalski, Leary, Blevins, & Holgate, 1997, Experiment 1).

More generally, various models suggest that affect influences how situations and persons are judged (see Forgas, 1992). For example, people in a sad mood (which is more typical for people with high, as opposed to low, depressive symptoms) attribute conflict more to internal, stable and global causes (Forgas, 1994), which, in turn, is likely to affect the perceived intensity of the conflict. Moreover, people in a sad mood identified more negative behaviour in videotaped interactions than people in a positive mood, and they recalled more details about difficult interactions later on (Forgas, Bower, & Krantz, 1984). Thus, mood-dependent effects have been found for attention as well as for memory, and these are likely to affect how conflicts are appraised.

Regarding secondary appraisal, a large body of research indicates that depressive symptoms are related to deficiencies in interpersonal competences such as conflict management (see Segrin, 2000). Thus, depressive symptoms predicted lower social skills in a non-clinical sample (Cole & Milstead, 1989). Coyne (1976) suggested that depressed people interact with others in a manner that is experienced as aversive by the interaction partners, for example, because the content of the conversation is negatively toned and self-referential. Furthermore, experimental laboratory studies suggest that people in a depressed mood tend to show more dysfunctional conflict behaviour (e.g. less cooperation, more competition) than people in a neutral mood (Forgas, 1998). Thus, people with high levels of depressive symptoms are likely to cope with conflicts less efficiently, which may cause conflicts to escalate. These negative effects may be further intensified by the fact that people with high levels of depressive symptoms are prone to ruminate about negative events and current feelings (Moulds, Kandris, Starr, & Wong, 2007; Nolen-Hoeksema, Morrow, & Fredrickson, 1993; Teasdale, 1983). Ruminative thoughts imply a continuing focus on stress appraisals, prolonging stress-related affective and physiological activations, and thus the duration of the negative effects of work stressors (see Brosschot, Gerin, & Thayer, 2006; Meurs & Perrewé, 2011). In line with this argument, the role of rumination has been stressed in the development of both depression (e.g. Nolen-Hoeksema, 1990) and somatic disease (e.g. Brosschot et al., 2006). All this suggests that people with high levels of depressive symptoms should react particularly strongly to conflicts at work.

The present study

Based on the considerations presented above, we suggest the following hypotheses:

Hypothesis 1: Interpersonal conflict will be negatively related to well-being.

Hypothesis 2: The effect of interpersonal conflict on well-being will be particularly strong among people with high levels of depressive symptoms.

Two considerations guided the selection of well-being indicators for our research. First, we wanted to include indicators of both psychological and physical well-being. Second, we wanted to ensure compatibility with existing research on conflict, and on stress more generally. With regard to psychological well-being, we followed the theory of subjective well-being by Diener, Oishi, and Lucas (2003), which includes affective and cognitive components. Furthermore, following Warr's (e.g. 1999, 2005) distinction between context-free and job-related well-being, we focused on *job-related* well-being and included job-related depressive mood as an indicator of the affective, and job satisfaction as indicator of the cognitive component. With regard to physical well-being, we used somatic complaints (Schat, Kelloway, & Desmarais, 2005) as an indicator. Importantly, all three outcomes have often been used as well-being indicators in previous research on conflict (e.g. Spector & Jex, 1998).

One may wonder why we chose depressive mood as an outcome while testing chronic depressive symptoms as moderator, as the two measures are conceptually very similar. However, it is absolutely conceivable that even the very same variable is an outcome of specific experiences (depressive tendencies are strengthened by conflict; cf. Dormann & Zapf, 1999) and a moderator at the same time (depressive tendencies are strengthened *more* for people who already have such tendencies to a relatively high degree, as their appraisal is particularly negative and their coping skills particularly poor). Note, however, that the outcome and the moderator were conceptualized differently in the present research.

In the first (cross-sectional) study, we focused on *job-related* depressive mood as outcome. Referring to one's work, job-related depressive mood is context-specific (Van Katwyk, Fox, Spector, & Kelloway, 2000); this distinguishes it from chronic depressive symptoms, which refer to a global negative feeling with self-destructive thoughts (see Stoner & Perrewé, 2006). When examining the effects of job-related stress on job-related depressive symptoms, it seems important to control for general depressive symptoms so it can be ruled out that effects found are due to a more general personal characteristic. Therefore, we examined whether interpersonal conflict was related to job-related depressive mood over and above the effect of general depressive symptoms, and if this effect was stronger for people high in general depressive symptoms, the latter referring to our discussion about the moderating role of depressive symptoms. Controlling for general depressive symptoms renders the test of both hypotheses rather rigorous, similar to controlling for negative affectivity in stress research (see Spector, Zapf, Chen, & Frese, 2000). In the second (diary) study, we focused on *state* depressive mood, assessed while people were at work. Thus, we examined if daily fluctuations in conflict have an effect on momentary depressive mood that cannot be explained by inter-individual differences in general depressive symptoms; again, we additionally tested if this effect was stronger for people high in general depressive symptoms.

By using these two different study designs, we were able to test the effect of conflict on well-being both at the inter-individual and at the intra-individual level. Most stress research tests if people experiencing more stressors (e.g. conflict) than other people will have a lower well-being than people experiencing fewer stressors, thus assessing between-person effects. In contrast, studies on intra-individual effects test if a person experiencing more stressors than usual will have lower well-being than usual, thus assessing within-person effects. Thus, the two analyses address related but distinct questions (see also Cervone, 2005).

Method

Method overview

To test our hypotheses, we conducted a cross-sectional and a diary study in Switzerland. In both studies, participants were recruited by research assistants via direct or indirect (e.g. email, phone) contact among their acquaintances. When interest in participating was expressed, the research assistants met the participants individually, explained the procedure and distributed the survey. However, the participants were not told which specific work condition and aspect of well-being would be measured. In the cross-sectional study, participants returned the survey with a prepaid envelope to the first author. In the diary study, the students kept contact (on average every other day) with the participants to answer any questions and to sustain the participants' commitment during data collection. Participants regularly returned their survey to the research assistants in sealed envelopes. As a compensation for the participants' time and as an incentive for their participation, participants were offered written individual feedback by the first author about their work situation and their well-being after the study was finished. If the results were critical, they were discussed with the participant in detail, advice was given on how to cope with work stress, and they were given web links to additional sources of help as well as the first author's contact information.

Study 1: Cross-sectional study

Participants and procedure

The sample consisted of 218 employees, holding a variety of jobs, such as shop assistant (30%), nurse (12%), administrative staff (12%) or software engineer (5%), plus various other occupations (mainly professionals such as lawyers and consultants). Blue-collar workers, such as cooks, were relatively rare (9%). Mean age was 35.7 years (SD = 11.4; range = 17–64). A slight majority (52%) was female. Forty-two per cent had completed regular school (9 years) or an apprenticeship, 35% had completed college and 23% had a university degree. All participants worked at least 50% of a full-time equivalent (FTE). Mean organizational tenure was 6.1 years (SD = 6.9; range = .1–35.0 years).

Measures

Conflict at work. Conflict was measured with the relationship conflict scale by Jehn (1995). The scale consisted of four items (e.g. "How often is there tension among

35

members in your work unit?"). The response format ranged from *very rarely/never* (1) to *very often/all the time* (5). Internal consistency was $\alpha = .91$.

General depressive symptoms. Chronic depressive symptoms were assessed with a short version of German version of the Center for Epidemiologic Studies Depression Scale (CES-D; Radloff, 1977; German version by Hautzinger & Bailer, 1993). The CES-D is a frequently employed measure for assessing depressive symptoms in nonclinical, subclinical and clinical populations (Eaton, Smith, Ybarra, Muntaner, & Tien, 2004). Participants were instructed to assess how frequently they had experienced each symptom within the preceding 30 days (e.g. "I felt depressed"). The scale consisted of 15 items. The answering format ranged from *seldom/not at all* (1) to *mostly* (4). Internal consistency was $\alpha = .93$.

Job-related depressive mood. Job-related depressive mood was assessed with five items from the Job-Related Affective Well-Being Scale (JAWS) by Van Katwyk et al. (2000) that focuses on negative evaluation and low arousal (e.g. depressed, gloomy). Participants had to indicate how often *their job made them feel* each emotion in the last 30 days. Response choice ranged from *never* (1) to *extremely often/always* (5). Internal consistency was $\alpha = .76$.

Job satisfaction. Job satisfaction was assessed with a scale by Baillod and Semmer (1994). The scale has four items, one of which is a Kunin Faces Scale asking "How satisfied are you in general with your work?". It ranges from *extremely dissatisfied* (1) to *extremely satisfied* (7). The other items ask participants to indicate how often they had specific thoughts about their work (e.g. "I hope my job situation will always remain as good as it is now"), ranging from *never* (1) to *always* (7). Internal consistency was $\alpha = .81$.

Somatic complaints. Somatic complaints were assessed with seven items about headaches and gastrointestinal problems from the Physical Health Questionnaire (PHQ) by Schat et al. (2005). Participants indicated how frequently they had experienced each symptom within the preceding 30 days on a Likert scale ranging from *never* (1) to *very often/all the time* (7). The sum of these items is a meaningful indicator of somatic complaints; however, it does not reflect a single underlying construct (see Schat et al., 2005). Therefore, internal consistency is not a meaningful measure for this scale (see Spector & Jex, 1998).

Confirmatory factor analyses

To ensure that our predictors and outcomes represented empirically distinguishable constructs, we conducted confirmatory factor analyses. Specifically, we examined whether a five-factor model was better than a one-factor model. The proposed five-factor model, containing conflict, general depressive symptoms, job-related depressive mood, somatic complaints and job satisfaction, had a good fit ($\chi^2(125) = 202.40$, Comparative Fit Index (CFI) = .97, Tucker-Lewis Index (TLI) = .96, root-mean-square error of approximation (RMSEA) = .06, standardized root mean squared residual (SRMR) = .06), which was significantly better than the fit for the one-factor model ($\chi^2(135) = 1167.31$, CFI = .56, TLI

= .50, RMSEA = .19, SRMR = .16; $\Delta\chi^2(10) = 964.91, p < .05$) and a four-factor model that combined chronic depressive symptoms and job-related depressive mood into a single factor ($\chi^2(129) = 306.54$, CFI = .92, TLI = .91, RMSEA = .08, SRMR = .07; $\Delta\chi^2(4) = 104.09, p < .05$). Additionally, we examined whether chronic depressive symptoms and job-related depressive mood were distinct constructs. A two-factor model had a good model fit ($\chi^2(19) = 43.40$, CFI = .98, TLI = .97, RMSEA = .08, SRMR = .04), which was significantly better than the fit of the one-factor model ($\chi^2(20) = 131.16$, CFI = .90, TLI = .86, RMSEA =.16, SRMR = .07; $\Delta\chi^2(1) = 87.76, p < .05$).

Control variables

Previous research has shown that women are more likely than men to experience depression (Nolen-Hoeksema, 1990), which may be the result of women's greater reactivity to stressors (see Nolen-Hoeksema, 2001) or of women's more frequent experience of interpersonal conflicts (e.g. Narayanan, Menon, & Spector, 1999). Furthermore, age is related to depression (e.g. Burke, Burke, Regier, & Rae, 1990); research suggests that older people are more likely to manage conflicts through problem solving (Van Lange, Otten, De Bruin, & Joireman, 1997), and to use more adaptive emotion regulation strategies (e.g. reappraisal; John & Gross, 2004) than younger people. Therefore, to test if the proposed interaction effect of conflicts and depressive symptoms was spurious, we controlled for gender and age.

Study 2: Diary study

Participants and procedure

The sample consisted of 127 employees holding a variety of jobs, such as administrative staff (22%), computer specialist (13%), social worker (7%), or engineer (6%), plus various other occupations (mainly professionals such as architects and consultants). Blue-collar workers, such as toolmakers were relatively rare (9%). Mean age was 35.6 years ($SD = 11.5$; range = 16–59 years). A slight majority (55%) was male. Thirty-two per cent had completed regular school (9 years) or an apprenticeship, 44% had completed college and 24% had a university degree. All of the participants worked at least 50% of a FTE. Organizational tenure ranged from 0.1 to 35.0 years; average tenure was 5.1 years ($SD = 6.7$).

Before the diary study started, participants completed a general questionnaire assessing their chronic level of depressive symptoms and demographic variables. At the beginning of the following week, participants began completing daily surveys for two weeks, including the weekend. To reduce the contamination of the predictor (conflict) by the outcome, we assessed the predictor and the outcome separately (see Ohly, Sonnentag, Niessen, & Zapf, 2010).. In the afternoon, approximately 1.5 hours before the end of work, participants filled out a questionnaire about positive and negative events at work (e. g. conflict). At the end of work, they reported their momentary well-being (i.e. depressive mood, job satisfaction, somatic complaints). On non-working days, participants were asked to omit the afternoon survey (assessing work events), but to fill out the end-of-work survey (assessing well-being).

Of the 127 participants in the initial sample, 58 did not report any working day with conflicts. Having no intra-individual variance in the predictor (i.e. conflict), these 58 participants were removed from the data set, yielding a final sample of

69 participants. Overall, they completed 603 afternoon surveys, corresponding to a mean of 8.6 (SD = 1.8) per participant, and 916 end-of-work surveys, corresponding to 13.3 (SD = 1.4) per participant. The participants who were excluded did not differ from the remaining ones with regard to gender, age and tenure. However, they reported fewer chronic depressive symptoms than those who were included (d = .58, p < .05). We see three possible reasons for this difference. First, the participants included experienced more conflicts, which can cause depression (see Hypothesis 1). Second, employees with higher levels of depressive symptoms may provoke more conflicts (e.g. Cummings, Hayes, Laurenceau, & Cohen, 2010). Third, employees with higher levels of depressive symptoms may perceive situations as more conflict-ridden (Beck, 1987). Note, however, that we centred conflict (a Level 1 variable) about the individual mean (group mean centring), which implies that all between-person variance was removed. Thus, the results cannot be interpreted in terms of stable differences between persons, and the coefficients for conflict reflect the effect of a person having many or few conflicts relative to his or her own mean for that variable across days. Nevertheless, we ran additional analyses with the complete sample (N = 127); results were almost identical (i.e. significant main effects and cross-level interaction effects of very similar size).

Measures

Conflict at work. Conflict at work was measured with a single item in the afternoon survey ("Today, I had a conflict at work"). The response format ranged from *completely disagree* (1) to *completely agree* (4).

State depressive mood. At the end of work, daily depressive mood was measured with a shortened five-item version of the CES-D (Radloff, 1977; see Study 1). We adapted the wording to refer to how participants felt during that day ("Today, I felt I could not shake off the blues"). The response format ranged from *completely disagree* (1) to *completely agree* (5). The reliability of the scale, calculated according to Nezlek (2007), was .73.

State job satisfaction. At the end of work, job satisfaction was measured using a single item ("How satisfied are you with your work at the moment?") with a faces scale (Kunin, 1955), consisting of seven faces, ranging from *extremely dissatisfied* (1) to *extremely satisfied* (7).

State somatic complaints. At the end of work, somatic complaints were assessed with four items from Mohr (1986), assessing headaches and gastrointestinal problems with two items each. Participants indicated how they felt at the moment (e.g. "At the moment, I have a headache"). The response format ranged from *completely disagree* (1) to *completely agree* (5). As noted above, internal consistency is not an appropriate indicator of reliability for this scale.

Chronic depressive symptoms. We used the same measure (CES-D; Radloff, 1977) as in Study 1. Internal consistency was .86.

Control variables. As in Study 1, we controlled for gender and age in our analyses.

Results

Cross-sectional study (Study 1)

Means, standard deviations and zero-order correlations are shown in Table 1. We conducted hierarchical regression analyses to test our hypotheses, centring predictor variables around their mean to facilitate the interpretation of main effects in models containing interaction terms (Aiken & West, 1991). We entered conflict and depressive symptoms in the first step, and their interaction in the second step. To examine the impact of the control variables, we entered age and gender in the third step, and the interaction of conflict and age, as well as the interaction of conflict and gender in the fourth step. However, the inclusion of age and gender did not alter the results. Therefore, we dropped the control variables from the final analyses. For directional hypotheses one-tailed tests were used.

Results of the hierarchical regression analyses are displayed in Table 2. In line with Hypothesis 1, conflict was related positively to job-related depressive mood and negatively to job satisfaction. Unexpectedly, conflict was not related to somatic complaints when we controlled for depressive symptoms. Note, however, that the bivariate correlation between conflict and somatic complaints was significant (see Table 1). Moreover, as postulated in Hypothesis 2, depressive symptoms had a strengthening effect on the slope

Table 1. Descriptive statistics and zero-order correlations of study variables in Study 1.

Variables	M	SD	1	2	3	4	5	6
1. Gender[a]	.48	–	–					
2. Age	35.67	11.38	.11	–				
3. Conflict	2.26	0.81	−.01	.04	–			
4. Chronic depressive symptoms	1.67	0.54	.05	−.11	.19*	–		
5. Job-related depressive mood	2.32	0.69	−.01	−.20*	.31*	.71*	–	
6. Job satisfaction	4.44	1.23	−.05	.10	−.32*	−.39*	−.51*	–
7. Somatic complaints	2.05	0.96	−.21*	−.16*	.14*	.51*	−.49*	−.33*

Note: $N = 218$. [a]0 = female, 1 = male. *$p < .05$.

Table 2. Hierarchical multiple regression analyses predicting job-related depressive mood, job satisfaction and somatic complaints (Study 1).

Predictor	Job-related depressive mood		Job satisfaction		Somatic complaints	
	ΔR^2	β	ΔR^2	β	ΔR^2	β
Step 1	.53*		.22*		.26*	
Conflict		.17*		−.26*		.04
Chronic depressive symptoms		.67*		−.34*		.50*
Step 2	.01*		.03*		.02*	
Conflict × Depressive symptoms		.10*		−.18*		.13*

Note: $N = 218$. *$p < .05$.

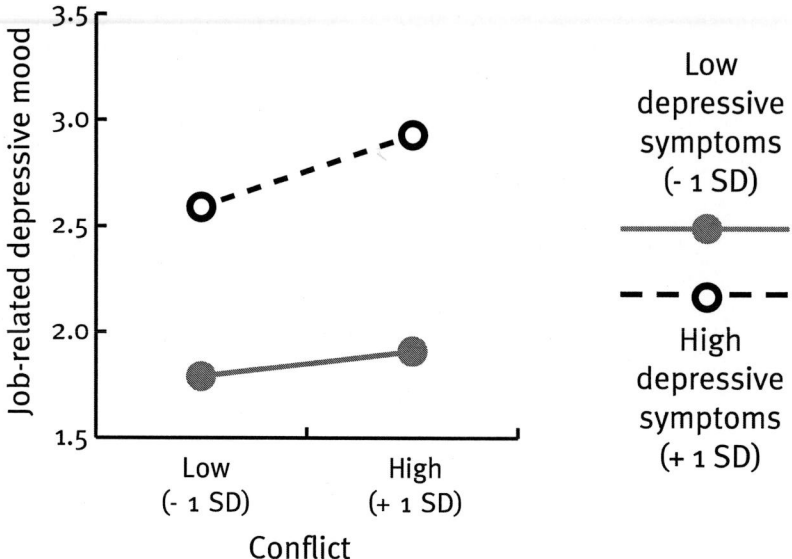

Figure 1. Interaction between conflict and chronic depressive symptoms predicting impaired well-being.

of conflict for depressive mood, job satisfaction and somatic complaints. For a more specific test of our hypotheses, we conducted simple slope tests for values 1 *SD* above and below the mean, as suggested by Aiken and West (1991). In line with our assumption, conflict was related to job-related depressive mood ($B = .21, p < .01$), job satisfaction ($B = -.58, p < .01$), and somatic complaints ($B = .16, p < .05$) only among people with relatively high levels of depressive symptoms, but not among people with low levels of depressive symptoms ($B = .07$, B $= -.12$, and $B = -.10$, respectively, all *ns*). Figure 1 illustrates these results for job-related depressive mood. The graphs for the other outcomes, not shown for reasons of space, were very similar and can be obtained from the first author.

Diary study (Study 2)

Data analysis

Because the daily data were nested within persons, we analyzed them with a multi-level random coefficient model, using the program HLM 6.06 (Raudenbush, Bryk, Cheong, & Congdon, 2004). We examined the within-person relations between conflict at work and well-being. To model the change in each outcome, we controlled for its baseline level by including the previous assessment as a predictor (i.e. well-being at the previous day). Level 1 predictors (conflict and baseline measures of the outcomes) were group mean-centred.

Of special interest was whether chronic depressive symptoms had an influence on the effect of daily conflict on state well-being. The measure of chronic depressive symptoms was centred around the grand mean to predict (i) the Level 1 intercept (i.e. the influence of chronic depressive symptoms on state well-being) and (ii) the Level 1 slope of conflict (i.e. the moderating effect of chronic depressive symptoms on the effect of conflict on state well-being). Furthermore, gender (uncentred), and age (grand-mean centred) were entered as covariates. However, with one exception that is noted, the inclusion of gender

Table 3.   Descriptive statistics and zero-order correlations of study variables in Study 2.

Variables	N	M	SD	ICC	1	2	3
Chronic measures (Level 2)							
1. Gender[a]	69	0.49	–	–	–	–	–
2. Age	69	35.41	10.85	–	.12	–	–
3. Chronic depressive symptoms	69	1.67	0.41	–	.07	.11	–
Daily measures (Level 1)							
1. Conflict	603	1.45	0.87	.04[b]	–		
2. Depressive mood	916	1.48	0.66	.38	.19*	–	
3. Job satisfaction	915	5.19	1.15	.53	−.13*	−.37*	–
4. Somatic complaints	906	1.21	0.41	.47	.05	.32*	−.11*

Note: Within-person (Level 1) correlations were calculated using the Mplus program (Muthén & Muthén, 2010). ICC = Intraclass correlation (proportion of the between-person variance compared with the total variance). [a]0 = female, 1 = male. [b]ICC of sample with unrestricted between-person variance in conflict (see Method section) is .15.
*$p < .05$.

and age did not alter the results. Therefore, the control variables were dropped from the final analyses. We used the restricted maximum-likelihood procedure in HLM to estimate the fixed and random parameters and the robust standard errors for the significance tests (see Hox, 2010). For directional hypotheses one-tailed tests were used.

Findings

Means, standard deviations, intra class correlations and zero-order correlations for the diary study are shown in Table 3. Results of the multilevel analyses are displayed in Table 4. In line with Hypothesis 1, conflict was positively related to state depressive mood and to state somatic complaints, and negatively related to state job satisfaction. Moreover, as postulated in Hypothesis 2, chronic depressive symptoms had a strengthening effect on the slope of conflict for all three outcome measures. For a more specific test of our hypotheses, we conducted simple slope tests using a tool by Preacher, Curran, and Bauer (2006). In line with our assumption, and replicating the findings from Study 1, conflict was related to state depressive mood ($B = .28, p < .01$), state job satisfaction ($B = −.34, p < .01$), and state somatic complaints ($B = .06, p < .05$) only among people with high, but not among people with low levels of chronic depressive symptoms ($B = .07, p < .05, B = −.08, ns$ and $B = .01, ns$, respectively). The result pattern was very similar to the one shown in Figure 1; graphs for these analyses can be obtained from the first author.

Discussion

This research showed that depressive symptoms strengthened the negative effect of conflict at work on psychological and physical well-being. More specifically, conflict was particularly strongly linked to job satisfaction, depressive mood and somatic complaints among people with high levels of depressive symptoms. This effect was found in both a cross-sectional and a diary study, and thus held for chronic conflict as well as for daily conflict, and at the between-person level as well as at the within-person level.

Table 4. Multilevel analyses predicting depressive mood, job satisfaction and somatic complaints (Study 2).

	Depressive mood		Job satisfaction		Somatic complaints	
	B	SE B	B	SE B	B	SE B
Intercept	1.47*	0.04	5.09*	0.09	1.19*	0.03
Effects of Level 1 variables						
Conflict	0.18*	0.03	−0.22*	0.07	0.04*	0.02
Autocorrelation	0.07	0.05	0.09*	0.05	0.08	0.06
Effects of chronic depressive symptoms on:						
Intercept	0.67*	0.08	−0.94*	0.20	0.25*	0.07
Slope of conflict	0.25*	0.06	−0.32*	0.16	$0.07^{\dagger a}$	0.05

Note: [a]In the model with age and sex as control variables, the effect was significant ($B = .09$, $p < .05$).
$^{\dagger}p < .10$. $*p < .05$.

The fact that conflict was negatively related to well-being is in line with previous research (see Spector & Bruk-Lee, 2008). The main contribution of the present study relates to the role of depressive symptoms as a *moderator*, which extends previous research. In line with our assumption, employees with higher levels of depressive symptoms reacted particularly strongly to conflict. These findings point to a potentially dangerous vicious circle: conflicts at work induce depressive mood, which in the long run makes people even more vulnerable to conflicts. This might be a central mechanism through which the experience of daily hassles such as conflicts, even if minor, may lead to more severe psychological problems (e.g. clinical depression), which cause suffering and impaired job performance (Adler et al., 2006), and can have economic cost implications (e.g. Greenberg et al., 2003; McTernan, Dollard, & LaMontagne, 2013). Note that depressive symptoms strengthened the effect of conflict not only on psychological but also on physical health. Thus, depressive symptoms are a vulnerability factor that is likely to undermine both psychological and physical resources. In a more general sense, such mechanisms could produce the "loss spirals" postulated by conservation of resources theory (Hobfoll, 2001).

Studies focusing on psychological well-being not only as an outcome but also as a moderator in the stressor-strain relationship are rare. The few studies indicating that well-being is a vulnerability factor have focused on physical well-being. Mulders, Meijman, O'Hanlon, and Mulder (1982) showed that bus drivers with high sickness frequency had stronger neuro-endocrine reactions at work than those with low sickness frequency. Similarly, Elfering, Grebner, Gerber, and Semmer (2008) showed that work stressors were particularly strongly related to norepinephrine excretion among people with high levels of musculoskeletal pain. Kottwitz et al. (2013) showed that perceived health moderated the association between illegitimate tasks and cortisol. Research on impaired *psychological* well-being as a vulnerability factor, however, is widely lacking, and we hope that the present study inspires scholars to consider (impaired) well-being not only as an outcome but also as an important part of the stress process. In terms of conservation of resources theory (e.g. Hobfoll, 2001), increased levels of depressive symptoms imply a loss of resources, which, in turn, increases vulnerability to further negative events.

In both studies, our outcomes included a variable that had a special relationship to our moderator, that is, depressive symptoms. Job-related depressive mood (Study 1) concerns a variable that is akin to depressive symptoms, albeit in a much more specific and circumscribed way; being tied more specifically to working conditions, it also is likely to be more malleable than general depressive symptoms. In Study 2, state depressive mood was assessed, which again is more specific and malleable than depressive symptoms in general. Such more specific well-being indicators are likely to be more reactive to working conditions than general depressive symptoms. In line with emotion-centred process models of job stress (e.g. Spector & Bruk-Lee, 2008) that propose that stressors such as conflict trigger negative emotions which then lead to more chronic strain, it is likely that (job-related and state) depressive mood feeds back into chronic depressive symptoms if it occurs frequently over an extended period. Such specific and more focused indicators of depressive mood may, therefore, be a mediator in the process through which conflict (and other stressors) may, in the long run, lead to yet higher depressive symptoms.

Practical implications

With regard to practical implications, our results highlight the importance of conditions at work. The present study focused on the interplay of individual differences and social conditions at work. Individual differences are traditionally in the focus of selection procedures, because they correlate with performance (e.g. Barrick, Mount, & Judge, 2001) or because they are related to the ability to cope with stressful conditions at work (as in the present study). However, focusing exclusively on selection would ignore the possibility that depressive symptoms may partly be an effect of working conditions that are characterized by conflict and interpersonal tensions (Dormann & Zapf, 1999). Our finding that the main effects explained more variance than the interaction effects suggests that it may be most promising to focus on working conditions in terms of minimizing conflict (e.g. foster trust and support and minimize tensions, see De Dreu & Van de Vliert, 1997; Folger, Poole, & Stutman, 2001). Additionally, stress reduction programmes based on redesigning jobs with lower job demands, and better conditions of cooperation and communication (e.g. Kawakami, Araki, Kawashima, Masumoto, & Hayashi, 1997) may be worth considering. Finally, training in coping skills (e.g. van der Klink, Blonk, Schene, & van Dijk, 2001) seems to be promising in reducing depressive symptoms. Furthermore, supervisors might be trained in recognizing depressive symptoms and in interpreting poor conflict behaviour as a sign of poor coping skills rather than in terms of hostile intentions, and they might be trained in fostering ways of dealing with conflicts that minimize threats to the sense of being accepted.

Certain limitations in the present study should be acknowledged. First, the idea of a vicious circle should be tested with longitudinal studies; they could clarify how long it takes until conflicts impact depressive symptoms, and they should try to replicate the moderating effect of depressive symptoms. They should also investigate the effect of more circumscribed and focused indicators of depressive symptoms, such as state depressive mood and job-related depressive mood, on the long-term development of depressive symptoms in a more general sense. Moreover, longitudinal studies would also shed further light on the role of depressive symptoms in predicting conflict. Researchers have proposed that conflict may be not only the cause but also the result of impaired well-being such as chronic depressive symptoms (e.g. De Dreu & Beersma, 2005). Recent findings from related research about justice (Lang, Bliese, Lang, & Adler, 2011) and bullying (Finne et al., 2011) suggests that chronic depressive symptoms may also lead to the experience of poorer work conditions (more injustice, more bullying). We found no support for such effects in Study 2; however, future research may use shorter timeframes (e.g. depressive mood in the morning and conflict during the same day) as well as longer ones (e.g. chronic depressive symptoms and chronic conflict over several months). It is important to note, however, that such reversed effects are not the same as the moderator effects presented here, nor can they explain these moderator effects. Reversed effects indicate that depressed people will experience, or generate, more conflicts than non-depressed people; the moderating effect indicates that a given amount of conflict is more strongly related to impaired well-being among people with more depressive symptoms than among people with fewer depressive symptoms.

Second, various scholars (e.g. Jehn, 1995) have suggested differentiating between two types of conflict, namely relationship conflict (interpersonal disagreement associated with feelings of animosity) and task conflict (disagreement about the best way to solve a problem). Whereas this distinction is common in research on performance, it has been largely ignored in research on well-being and stress (Spector & Bruk-Lee, 2008). The existing studies, however, have consistently found negative associations between relationship conflict and well-being; the pattern is less clear for task conflict (see Meier et al., 2013). Given that relationship conflict is more strongly related to feelings of rejection than task conflict (e.g. De Dreu, Harinck, & Van Vianen, 1999), it is possible that the increased vulnerability of people with high levels of depressive symptoms is restricted to relationship conflict. In the current paper, we focused on relationship conflict in the cross-sectional study; in the diary study we used a single item, which does not allow conclusions about the type of conflict. We therefore could not examine the moderating role of depressive symptoms for relationship and task conflict separately, and we suggest such analyses for future research.

Third, the present study did not test the potential mechanism of why people with high levels of depressive symptoms reacted more strongly to conflict. As an example, we postulated that conflicts are threatening the need to belong and therefore are more stressful for individuals with high levels of depressive symptoms because of their insecure feelings of belonging and fears of abandonment. Future research could therefore examine whether the effect of conflict on strain is mediated by a threatened need to belong and how depressive symptoms moderates this indirect relation (i.e. moderated mediation tests). As a second example, we noted that individuals with high levels of depressive symptoms show lower conflict management skills, which may cause conflicts to escalate. Future studies could therefore examine the degree to which the moderating effect of depressive symptoms can be explained by differences in conflict management style (i.e. mediated moderation tests). In general, future research should focus more on the underlying mechanism to inform theory and practice about the increased vulnerability of people with high levels of depressive symptoms.

Finally, both studies used a convenience sample, which imposes limits on general-izability. More specifically, our samples were rather highly educated, which may imply comparatively low reactivity to stressors in general, and to conflicts in particular (see, for instance, Almeida, 2005). Our findings should be replicated using samples more representative of the employed population.

Conclusions

Our findings from both a cross-sectional survey and a diary study indicate that chronic depressive symptoms are a vulnerability factor to work stress in the form of interpersonal conflict at work. In line with previous research, both enduring conflicts and daily conflicts were negatively related to both psychological and physical well-being. These effects were particularly strong for employees with impaired psychological resources, namely those with relatively high levels of depressive symptoms. Thus, conflicts may cause depressive symptoms, which in turn make people even more vulnerable to conflicts, indicating a vicious circle with high psychological costs to the individual and economic costs to the organization.

Funding

This research was supported in part by Grants [PA001-131482] and [PZ00P1-142393] from the Swiss National Science Foundation to Laurenz L. Meier.

References

Adler, D., McLaughlin, T., Rogers, W., Chang, H., Lapitsky, L., & Lerner, D. (2006). Job performance deficits due to depression. *American Journal of Psychiatry, 163*, 1569–1576.

Aiken, L. S., & West, S. G. (1991). *Multiple regression: Testing and interpreting interactions.* Newbury Park, CA: Sage.

Almeida, D. (2005). Resilience and vulnerability to daily stressors assessed via diary methods. *Current Directions in Psychological Science, 14*(2), 64–68.

Baillod, J., & Semmer, N. (1994). Fluktuation und Berufsverläufe bei Computerfachleuten [Turnover and career paths of computer specialists]. *Zeitschrift für Arbeits- und Organisationspsychologie, 38*, 152–163.

Baldwin, G., & Shean, G. D. (2006). A taxometric study of the Center for Epidemiological Studies Depression Scale. *Genetic, Social, and General Psychology Monographs, 132*, 101–128.

Barrick, M. R., Mount, M. K., & Judge, T. A. (2001). Personality and performance at the beginning of the new millennium: What do we know and where do we go next? *International Journal of Selection and Assessment, 9*, 9–30.

Baumeister, R. F., & Leary, M. R. (1995). The need to belong: Desire for interpersonal attachments as a fundamental human motivation. *Psychological Bulletin, 11*, 497–529.

Beck, A. T. (1987). Cognitive models of depression. *Journal of Cognitive Psychotherapy, 1*, 5–37.

Blatt, S., Quinlan, D. M., Chevron, E. S., McDonald, C., & Zuroff, D. (1982). Dependancy and self-criticism: Psychological dimensions of depression. *Journal of Consulting and Clinical Psychology, 50*(1), 113–124.

Burke, K. C., Burke, J. D., Regier, D. A., & Rae, D. S. (1990). Age at the onset of selected mental-disorders in five community populations. *Archives of General Psychiatry, 47*, 511–518.

Bolger, N., DeLongis, A., Kessler, R. C., & Schilling, A. (1989). Effects of daily stress on negative mood. *Journal of Personality and Social Psychology, 57*, 808–818.

Bonde, J. P. E. (2008). Psychosocial factors at work and risk of depression: A systematic review of the epidemiological evidence. *Occupational and Environmental Medicine, 65*, 438–445.

Brosschot, J., Gerin, W., & Thayer, J. (2006). The perseverative cognition hypothesis: A review of worry, prolonged stress-related physiological activation, and health. *Journal of Psychosomatic Research, 60*(2), 113–124.

Cervone, D. (2005). Personality architecture: Within-person structures and processes. *Annual Review of Psychology, 56*, 423–452.

Cole, D. A., & Milstead, M. (1989). Behavioral correlates of depression: Antecedents or consequences? *Journal of Counseling Psychology, 36*, 408–416.

Coyne, J. C. (1976). Depression and the response of others. *Journal of Abnormal Psychology, 85*, 186–193.

Cummings, J. A., Hayes, A. M., Laurenceau, J.-P., & Cohen, L. H. (2010). Conflict management mediates the relationship between depressive symptoms and daily negative events: Interpersonal competence and daily stress generation. *International Journal of Cognitive Therapy*, *3*, 318–331.

De Dreu, C., & Beersma, B. (2005). Conflict in organizations: Beyond effectiveness and performance. *European Journal of Work and Organizational Psychology*, *14*(2), 105–117.

De Dreu, C. K. W., & Gelfand, M. J. (2008). Conflict in the workplace: Sources, functions, and dynamics across multiple levels of analysis. In C. K. W. De Dreu & M. J. Gelfand (Eds.), *The psychology of conflict and conflict management in organizations* (pp. 3–54). New York, NY: Lawrence Erlbaum.

De Dreu, C. K. W., Harinck, F., & Van Vianen, A. E. M. (1999). Conflict and performance in groups and organizations. In C. L. Cooper & I. T. Robertson (Eds.), *International review of industrial and organizational psychology* (Vol. 144, pp. 369–414). Chichester: Wiley.

De Dreu, C. K. W., & Van de Vliert, E. (1997). *Using conflict in organizations*. London: Sage.

Diener, E., Oishi, S., & Lucas, R. E. (2003). Personality, culture, and subjective well-being: Emotional and cognitive evaluations of life. *Annual Review of Psychology*, *54*, 403–425.

Dormann, C., & Zapf, D. (1999). Social support, social stressors at work, and depressive symptoms: Testing for main and moderating effects with structural equations in a three-wave longitudinal study. *Journal of Applied Psychology*, *84*, 874–884.

Eaton, W. W., Smith, C., Ybarra, M., Muntaner, C., Tien, A. (2004). Center for Epidemiologic Studies Depression Scale: Review and revision (CESD and CESD-R). In M. E. Maruish (Ed.), *The use of psychological testing for treatment planning and outcomes assessment: Volume 3 (Instruments for adults)* (pp. 363–377). Mahwah, NJ: Erlbaum.

Elfering, A., Grebner, S., Gerber, H., & Semmer N. K. (2008). Workplace observation of work stressors, catecholamines and musculoskeletal pain among male employees. *Scandinavian Journal of Work and Environmental Health*, *34*, 337–344.

Ellsworth, P. C., & Scherer, K. R. (2003). Appraisal processes in emotion. In R. J. Davidson, K. R. Scherer, & H. Hill Goldsmith (Eds.), *Handbook of affective sciences* (pp. 572–595). Oxford: Oxford University Press.

Finne, L. B., Knardahl, S., & Lau, B. (2011). Workplace bullying and mental distress – a prospective study of Norwegian employees. *Scandinavian Journal of Work and Environmental Health*, *37*, 276–286.

Folger, J. P., Poole, M. S., & Stutman, R. K. (2001). *Working through conflict: Strategies far relationships, groups and organizations* (3rd ed.). New York: Addison, Wesley, Longman.

Forgas, J. P. (1992). Affect in social judgments and decisions: A multiprocess model. In M. P. Zanna (Ed.). *Advances in Experimental Social Psychology* (Vol. 25, pp. 227–275). New York, NY: Academic Press.

Forgas, J. P. (1994). Sad and guilty? Affective influences on the explanation of conflict in close relationships. *Journal of Personality and Social Psychology*, *66*(1), 56–68.

Forgas, J. (1998). On feeling good and getting your way: Mood effects on negotiator cognition and bargaining strategies. *Journal of Personality and Social Psychology*, *74*(3), 565–577.

Forgas, J. P., Bower, G. H., & Krantz, S. E. (1984). The influence of mood on perceptions of social interactions. *Journal of Experimental Social Psychology*, *20*, 497–513.

Greenberg, P., Kessler, R., Birnbaum, H., Leong, S., Lowe, S., Berglund, P., & Corey-Lisle, P. K. (2003). The economic burden of depression in the United States: How did it change between 1990 and 2000? *Journal of Clinical Psychiatry*, *64*, 1465–1475.

Hautzinger, M., & Bailer, M. (1993). *Allgemeine Depressions-Skala (ADS): Manual* [Center for Epidemiologic Studies Depression Scale (CES-D): Manual]. Weinheim: Beltz.

Hobfoll, S. E. (2001). The influence of culture, community, and the nested-self in the stress process: Advancing conservation of resources theory. *Applied Psychology: An International Review*, *50*, 337–421.

Hox, J. (2010). *Multilevel analysis. Techniques and applications* (2nd ed.). New York, NY: Routledge.

Ilies, R., Johnson, M. D., Judge, T. A., & Keeney, J. (2011). A within-individual study of interpersonal conflict as a work stressor: Dispositional and situational moderators. *Journal of Organizational Behavior*, *32*(1), 44–64.

Jehn, K. A. (1995). A multimethod examination of the benefits and detriments of intragroup conflict. *Administrative Science Quarterly*, *40*, 256–285.

John, O. P., & Gross, J. J. (2004). Healthy and unhealthy emotion regulation: Personality processes, individual differences, and life span development. *Journal of Personality, 72*, 1301–1334.

Kawakami, N., Araki, S., Kawashima, M., Masumoto, T., & Hayashi, T. (1997). Effects of work-related stress reduction on depressive symptoms among Japanese blue-collar workers. *Scandinavian Journal of Work, Environment and Health, 23*, 54–59.

Kottwitz, M. U., Meier, L. L., Jacobshagen, N., Kälin, W., Elfering, A., Hennig, J., & Semmer, N. K. (2013). Illegitimate tasks associated with higher cortisol levels among male employees when subjective health is relatively low: An intra-individual analysis. *Scandinavian Journal of Work, Environment and Health, 39*, 310–318.

Kunin, T. (1955). The construction of a new type of attitude measure. *Personnel Psychology, 8*, 66–77.

Lang, J., Bliese, P. D., Lang, J. W. B., & Adler, A. B. (2011). Work gets unfair for the depressed: Cross-lagged relations between organizational justice perceptions and depressive symptoms. *Journal of Applied Psychology, 96*, 602–618.

Lazarus, R. S. (1991). *Emotion and adaption*. New York, NY: Oxford University Press.

McTernan, W. P., Dollard, M. F. and LaMontagne, A. D. (2013). Depression in the workplace: An economic cost analysis of depression-related productivity loss attributable to job strain and bullying. *Work & Stress, 27*, 321–328.

Meier, L. L., Gross, S., Spector, P. E., & Semmer, N. K. (2013). Task and relationship conflict at work: Interactive short-term effects on angry mood and somatic complaints. *Journal of Occupational Health Psychology, 18*, 144–156.

Meurs, J. A., & Perrewe, P. L. (2011). Cognitive activation theory of stress: An integrative theoretical approach to work stress. *Journal of Management, 37*, 1043–1066.

Mohr, G. (1986). *Die Erfassung psychischer Befindensbeinträchtigungen bei Arbeitern* [The measurement of mental deterioration of blue-collar workers]. Frankfurt: Peter Lang.

Moulds, M. L., Kandris, E., Starr, S., & Wong, A. C. M. (2007). The relationship between rumination, avoidance and depression in a non-clinical sample. *Behaviour Research and Therapy, 45*, 251–261.

Mulders, H. P. G., Meijman, T. F., O'Hanlon, J. F., & Mulder, G. (1982). Differential psychophysiological reactivity of city bus drivers. *Ergonomics, 25*, 1003–1011.

Muthén, L. K., & Muthén, B. O. (2010). *Mplus user's guide* (6th ed.). Los Angeles, CA: Muthén & Muthén.

Narayanan, L., Menon, S., & Spector, P. (1999). Stress in the workplace: A comparison of gender and occupations. *Journal of Organizational Behavior, 20*(1), 63–73.

Nezlek, J. B. (2007). Multilevel modeling in research on personality. In R. Robins, R. C. Fraley, & R. Krueger (Eds.), *Handbook of research methods in personality psychology* (pp. 502–523). New York, NY: Guilford.

Nezlek, J. B., Kowalski, R. M., Leary, M. R., Blevins, T., & Holgate, S. (1997). Personality moderators of reactions to interpersonal rejection: Depression and trait self-esteem. *Personality and Social Psychology Bulletin, 23*, 1235–1244.

Nolen-Hoeksema, S. (1990). *Sex differences in depression*. Stanford, CA: Stanford University Press.

Nolen-Hoeksema, S. (2001). Gender differences in depression. *Current Directions in Psychological Science, 10*, 173–176.

Nolen-Hoeksema, S., Morrow, J., & Fredrickson, B. L. (1993). Response styles and the duration of episodes of depressed mood. *Journal of Abnormal Psychology, 102*, 20–28.

Ohly, S., Sonnentag, S., Niessen, C., & Zapf, D. (2010). Diary studies in organizational research. An introduction and some practical recommendations. *Journal of Personnel Psychology, 9*(2), 79–93.

Preacher, K., Curran, P., & Bauer, D. (2006). Computational tools for probing interactions in multiple linear regression, multilevel modeling, and latent curve analysis. *Journal of Educational and Behavioral Statistics, 31*, 437–448.

Prisciandaro, J., & Roberts, J. (2005). A taxometric investigation of unipolar depression in the national comorbidity survey. *Journal of Abnormal Psychology, 114*, 718–728.

Radloff, L. S. (1977). The CES-D Scale: A self-report depression scale for research in the general population. *Applied Psychological Measurement, 1*, 385–401.

Raudenbush, S. W., Bryk, A. S., Cheong, Y. K., & Congdon, R. T., Jr. (2004). *HLM 6: Hierarchical linear and nonlinear modeling* (Ver. 6.06). Lincolnwood, IL: Scientific Software International.

Ruscio, J., & Ruscio, A. (2000). Informing the continuity controversy: A taxometric analysis of depression. *Journal of Abnormal Psychology, 109*, 473–487.

Schat, A. C. H., Kelloway, E. K., & Desmarais, S. (2005). The Physical Health Questionnaire (PHQ): Construct validation of a self-report scale of somatic symptoms. *Journal of Occupational Health Psychology, 10*, 363–381.

Segrin, C. (2000). Social skills deficits associated with depression. *Clinical Psychology Review, 20*, 379–403.

Spector, P. E., & Bruk-Lee V. (2008). Conflict, health, and well-being. In C. K. W. De Dreu, & M. J. Gelfand (Eds.). *The psychology of conflict and conflict management in organizations* (pp. 267–288). San Francisco: Jossey-Bass.

Spector, P. E., & Jex, S. M. (1998). Development of four self-report measures of job stressors and strain: Interpersonal conflict at work scale, organizational constraints scale, quantitative workload inventory, and physical symptoms inventory. *Journal of Occupational Health Psychology, 3*, 356–367.

Spector, P. E., Zapf, D., Chen, P. Y., & Frese, M. (2000). Why negative affectivity should not be controlled in job stress research: don't throw out the baby with the bath water. *Journal of Organizational Behavior, 21*(1), 79–95.

Stoner, J., & Perrewé, P. L. (2006). The consequences of depressed mood at work: The influence of supportive supervisors, In A. M. Rossi, P. L. Perrewé, & S. L. Sauter (Eds.), *Current perspectives in occupational stress* (pp. 87–99). Greenwich: Information Age.

Teasdale, J. D. (1983). Negative thinking in depression: Cause, effect, or reciprocal relationship? *Advances in Behaviour Research and Therapy, 5*(1), 3–25.

Tennant, C. (2001). Work-related stress and depressive disorders. *Journal of Psychosomatic Research, 51*, 697–704.

Van der Klink, J. J. L., Blonk, R. W. B., Schene, A. H., & Van Dijk, F. J. H. (2001). The benefits of interventions for work-related stress. *American Journal of Public Health, 91*, 270–271.

Van Katwyk, P. T., Fox, S., Spector, P. E., & Kelloway, E. K. (2000). Using the Job-Related Affective Well-Being Scale (JAWS) to investigate affective responses to work stressors. *Journal of Occupational Health Psychology, 5*, 219–230.

Van Lange, P., Otten, W., De Bruin, E., & Joireman, J. (1997). Development of prosocial, individualistic, and competitive orientations: Theory and preliminary evidence. *Journal of Personality and Social Psychology, 73*, 733–746.

Warr, P. (1999). Well-being and the workplace. In D. Kahneman, E. Diener, & N. Schwarz (Eds.), *Well-being: The foundations of hedonic psychology* (pp. 392–412). New York, NY: Russell Sage Foundation.

Warr, P. (2005). Work, well-being, and mental health. In J. Barling, E. K. Kelloway, & M. R. Frone (Eds.), *Handbook of work stress* (pp. 547–574). Thousand Oaks, CA: Sage.

Ylipaavalniemi, J., Kivimäki, M., Elovainio, M., Virtanen, M., Keltikangas-Järvinen, L., & Vahtera, J. (2005). Psychosocial work characteristics and incidence of newly diagnosed depression: a prospective cohort study of three different models. *Social Science & Medicine, 61*(1), 111–122.

Enjoyment and absorption: An electronic diary study on daily flow patterns

Alma M. Rodríguez-Sánchez[a], Wilmar Schaufeli[b], Marisa Salanova[a], Eva Cifre[a]
and Mieke Sonnenschein[b]

[a]WoNT Research Team, Universitat Jaume I, Castellón, Spain; [b]Department of Psychology,
Utrecht University, Utrecht, The Netherlands

Flow experience is a state of mind in which one is totally absorbed in a task. This study explored the daily flow patterns related to working and non-working tasks among healthy and non-healthy (burned-out) individuals using the Experience Sampling Method. Previously the flow experience has been measured in terms of high challenges and high skills. The main aim of this study was to explore flow throughout the day using an operationalization that focused on the flow experience itself, as indicated by enjoyment and absorption. Forty healthy participants and 60 burned-out individuals kept an electronic diary on activities (work/non-work), and levels of flow (enjoyment and absorption) for 14 days. Entries were prompted by a signal on average five times a day, thus rendering 5455 entries. A curvilinear daily flow pattern was observed, with lower levels of flow during working hours. Differences were found between the components of flow: enjoyment was higher during non-working tasks, whereas absorption was higher when working. There were no differences in flow patterns between the healthy and burned-out group although the actual levels differed, with the former experiencing more flow than the latter. The results confirm the validity of this means of measuring flow, using enjoyment and absorption as indicators.

Introduction

The phenomenon of "flow" has captured the attention of a growing number of researchers since Csikszentmihalyi introduced the concept in the mid 1970s (Csikszentmihalyi, 1975). He interviewed artists, athletes, composers and scientists, and asked them to describe the "optimal experiences" that made them feel good and motivated as they were doing something that was worth doing for its own sake. He coined this experience "flow" because many interviewees used this term spontaneously to explain what their optimal experience felt like (Csikszentmihalyi & Csikszentmihalyi, 1988). Thus, flow is a condition in which people are so involved in an activity that nothing else seems to matter at the time, and the experience is so enjoyable that people will do it even at great cost for the sheer sake of doing it (Csikszentmihalyi, 1990).

Although the concept of flow may seem to be clear at the first glance, some problems exist in operationalizing the construct. This is mainly due to the difficulty of assessing or "capturing" the flow experience itself, as if momentary and experience. Because this "volatile" nature is inherent to flow, it is difficult to discriminate between the proximal antecedents and the flow experience itself. This also complicates the operationalization of flow. Traditionally, the flow experience has been measured in terms of the combination (i.e. product) of high challenges and high skills (Csikszentmihalyi & Lefevre, 1989; Delespaul, Reis, & deVries, 2004; Delle Fave, Bassi, & Massimini, 2003; Eisenberger, Jones, Stinglhamber, Shanock, & Randall, 2005). Namely, "when both challenges and skills are high, the person is not only enjoying the moment, but also stretching his or her capabilities with the likelihood of learning new skills and increasing self-esteem and personal complexity. This process of optimal experience has been called flow" (Csikszentmihalyi & Lefevre, 1989, p. 816). So, according to Csikszentmihalyi and Lefevre (1989) perceived challenge and skills are both antecedents of flow and constitute the experience itself. More recently, Nakamura and Csikszentmihalyi (2002) concur with this view and state that a match of high perceived skills and high challenges is a necessary – but not in itself sufficient – prerequisite to the experience of flow. However, how can flow in everyday life best be measured? In terms of prerequisites (the combination of high challenges and high skills), or in terms of a momentary experience? We decided on the latter because for our study, the main purpose of which was to explore daily patterns of flow, it was crucial to identify the flow experience itself and to distinguish it from its proximal antecedents (i.e. the match of high challenges with high skills).

The nature of flow

A review of the literature reveals that all definitions of flow experience seem to have three elements in common. The first refers to a sense of deep involvement and total concentration, in other words, *absorption* (Chen, 2006; Csikszentmihalyi, 1975; Ghani & Deshpande, 1994; Lutz & Guiry, 1994; Moneta & Csikszentmihalyi, 1996; Trevino & Webster, 1992). A second common element involves the positive feeling of enjoyment while being engaged in the activity, in other words *enjoyment* (Ghani & Deshpande, 1994; Hedman & Sharafi, 2004; Moneta & Csikszentmihalyi, 1996; Privette & Bundrick, 1987). The final element specifically refers to the interest in performing the activity for its own sake and not because of external demands or pressures, in other words *intrinsic interest*. (Moneta & Csikszentmihalyi, Salanova, Bakker, & Llorens, 2006; Trevino & Webster, 1992). In our view, rather than a constituting element of flow, intrinsic interest might act as an additional antecedent or prerequisite of the flow experience itself (Rodríguez-Sánchez, Cifre, Salanova, & Åborg, 2008). Furthermore, conceptually speaking, intrinsic interest should be conceived as a motivational factor that drives a person to engage in a particular intrinsically rewarding activity. By doing so, the likelihood of experiencing flow is increased. However, during the flow experience itself, intrinsic interest is not experienced. Hence, for empirical and conceptual reasons we limit the flow experience to enjoyment and absorption, thereby excluding intrinsic interest (cf. Chen, 2006; Csikszentmihalyi, 1990; Ghani & Deshpande, 1994). More specifically, enjoyment is considered to be the emotional component of flow and absorption its cognitive component.

Flow in healthy and non-healthy individuals

As the flow experience is positive by its very nature, it is plausible that "healthy" individuals are more likely to experience flow than "non-healthy" individuals. Perhaps for that reason previous research on flow typically used healthy samples. Note that in the present study we employed the term "healthy" to refer to individuals (in our case employees) who were neither on sick leave nor suffered from mental or physical illness. However, by way of comparison we also used a non-healthy, burned-out group. In doing so, we were able to investigate the implicit claim of previous flow studies that flow experiences are mainly found in healthy individuals. Burnout is defined as a chronic, work-related stress reaction characterized by exhaustion (i.e. fatigue due to excessive work demands), cynicism (i.e. indifferent, detached and distant attitudes towards one's work) and a lack of professional efficacy (i.e. the tendency to evaluate one's work negatively and feel incompetent) (Maslach, Schaufeli, & Leiter, 2001). However, there is accumulating evidence that exhaustion and cynicism constitute the core components of burnout (Schaufeli & Taris, 2005). In addition, we expected to find differences between flow in the healthy and the burned-out employees, since burnout is the opposite of engagement, which is closely related to (but not the same as) flow. More specifically, engagement represents a more long-term, positive work-related experience that bears some similarity to flow at work (Demerouti, 2006). Engagement is defined as a positive, fulfilling, work-related state of mind that is characterized by vigour, dedication and absorption. Besides, engagement refers to a persistent, pervasive and positive affective-motivational state of fulfilment in employees that does not focus on any particular object, event, individual or behaviour (Schaufeli, Salanova, González-Romá, & Bakker, 2002). The difference between work engagement and flow is that the former is a more general and pervasive work-related state of mind, whereas the latter is a more specific optimal experience of limited duration that relates to a specific objective (i.e. activity).

Therefore, since flow is a positive psychological state that is constituted by enjoyment and absorption, it is plausible that flow is negatively related to burnout, as conceived by exhaustion and cynicism. For instance, it is difficult to imagine that a burned-out employee, who is cynical and doubts the significance of his or her work, will experience flow, which is characterized by the opposite experiences such as enjoyment and absorption. Therefore, in our study we expected that:

Hypothesis 1. Flow levels will be significantly higher in healthy individuals as compared to non-healthy (burned-out) individuals.

Daily fluctuations in flow

Research into the dynamics of daily fluctuations of flow experiences is scarce. In fact, most previous studies have related flow experiences across the day to particular activities, such as studying, doing homework, socializing, arts and hobbies (e.g. Carli, Delle Fave, & Massimini, 1988; Massimini & Carli, 1988). But how does flow *fluctuate* across the day? As far as we know, only Guastello, Johnson, and Rieke (1999) paid attention to fluctuations of flow across time, and found that flow fluctuated in a non-linear dynamic fashion over a period of one week. However, no information exists about whether flow experiences follow a daily pattern that is associated with a specific activity. More particularly, it is not clear whether or not experiencing flow is related to the time of the day (i.e. follow a daily pattern analogously to the circadian rhythm) or to a particular work or leisure activity, irrespective of the time of the day. All we know so far is that flow is related to challenging activities.

Because flow includes an affective component (enjoyment), the literature on daily fluctuations of emotions might be helpful in understanding patterns of flow across time. Research shows that emotions exhibit non-linear rather than linear patterns of change in diurnal (e.g. Murray, Allen, Trinder, & Burgess, 2002; Rusting & Larsen, 1998) and weekly cycles (e.g. Larsen & Kasimatis, 1990). Most likely, the reason for this is that human emotions follow diurnal biological rhythms. For instance, Clark, Watson, and Leeka (1989) found that various indicators of positive affect rose sharply from early morning until noon; they remained relatively constant until 9 p.m., and then fell rapidly. Murray (2007) found similar results suggesting that positive affect displayed a diurnal rhythm in which a quadratic wave form was most prominent, consistent with the presence of a circadian component, typically experienced as a positive mood variation with mood being worse upon waking and better in the evening (Boivin et al., 1997; Koorengevel, Beersma, Gordjin, den Boer, & van den Hoofdakker, 2000). These results suggest that positive affect follows a diurnal rhythm and shows a non-linear pattern characterized by an inverted U-shape. It seems that the typical quadratic wave form found in diurnal positive affect under normal sleep-wake conditions can be understood as a segment of the 24-hour circadian rhythm (Clark et al., 1989).

Since our conceptualization of flow also includes a cognitive component (i.e. absorption) research on circadian rhythms in human cognition is of relevance too. For instance, Schmidt, Collette, Cajochen, and Peigneux (2007) observed that time-of-day modulations impacted on the performance of several cognitive tasks, and that these performance fluctuations were additionally contingent upon inter-individual differences in the circadian preference. Besides, that study found that some cognitive processes were particularly sensitive to variations at the circadian arousal level, whereas others were less affected.

Based on the diurnal variation found in positive affect and some cognitive processes, we hypothesize that:

Hypothesis 2. The flow experience will be related to time of day according to a diurnal pattern characterized by inverted U-shape.

In the same way as the time of the day may influence positive affect and certain cognitive processes, weekly fluctuations may have an effect on flow experiences too. In addition, fluctuations in positive affect also appear to relate with the day of the week and the season of the year (e.g. Rossi & Rossi, 1977; Smith, 1979; Stone, Hedges, Neale, & Satin, 1985). Weekly fluctuations might be influenced by the type of activities that individuals are carrying out. In other words, the activities in which people engage on weekdays differ from weekend activities. For instance, people work during weekdays and have more free time during the weekends. Therefore, the combination of the type of activity and the day of the week may influence in the likelihood of experiencing flow. Besides, flow tends to occur in challenging activities that require high levels of personal skills. In fact, people tend to experience more flow during work than in leisure activities, since using one's skills in a challenging situation is difficult to achieve outside work (Csikszentmihalyi & LeFevre, 1989). Thus, in order to clarify whether flow fluctuations are due not only to the type of activity but also due to the day of the week, in the present study we also explore differences in flow between weekdays and weekends. Hence, we hypothesize that:

> *Hypothesis 3*. Levels of flow will tend to be higher on weekdays as compared to weekends.

Flow in working and non-working tasks

It has been observed that individuals report more flow experiences during work than off-work, but at the same time – and paradoxically – they prefer leisure above work. This is known as the "paradox of work" (Csikszentmihalyi, 1990): work is likely to provoke more flow experiences than leisure, but leisure is preferred above work. During work people tend to take on more challenging activities than during leisure (Csikszentmihalyi & LeFevre, 1989). Besides, there is evidence for a positive relationship between flow experiences and high positive activation (Larsen & Diener, 1992; Russell & Carroll, 1999), which is more frequently observed at work than during leisure. So not surprisingly, it has been found that flow scores are higher during work, but scores for happiness or satisfaction are higher during leisure time (Rheinberg, Manig, Kliegl, Engeser, & Vollmeyer, 2007). Then, what is the reason for the paradox of preferring leisure activities over work, even though it provides more flow experiences? Since we operationalized flow in terms of two dimensions – enjoyment (affective) and absorption (cognitive), we are able to study this paradox in greater detail. Namely, on the one hand, we expected that particularly levels of enjoyment would be higher in non-working tasks as compared to working tasks. On the other hand, working tasks are by definition goal-directed and usually include cognitive processes that require concentration and a certain amount of absorption (Schmidt et al., 2007). Or put differently, "concentration" (Schallberger & Pfister, 2001) – or absorption in our terms – is more characteristic of working activities than of non-working activities. Thus, we expect that:

> *Hypothesis 4*. Enjoyment will be positively related to non-working tasks, whereas absorption is positively related to working tasks.

Finally, since there is no *a priori* reason why "healthy" and "non-healthy" individuals would differ in terms of their daily patterns of flow experiences, we hypothesized that:

> *Hypothesis 5*. The daily patterns of flow experiences will be similar for healthy and non-healthy (burned-out) individuals.

Note that whereas this hypothesis refers to *patterns*, Hypothesis 1 assumes that the *levels* of flow differ between healthy and non-healthy individuals.

Method

Participants

The participants were 40 healthy individuals (Mean age = 41.8, $SD = 10.0$: 65% females; 65% educated at college/university) from different occupational groups, and 60 clinically burned-out individuals (Mean age = 42.9, $SD = 8.8$: 55% females; 58% educated at college/university). Healthy participants were recruited through newspaper advertisements (25%) and personal contacts (75%). In order to be labelled "healthy", participants had to score below the validated cut-off points for burnout (Schaufeli, Bakker, Hoogduin, Schaap, & Kladler, 2001) on the Dutch version of the Maslach Burnout Inventory – General Survey (MBI-GS) (Schaufeli & Van Dierendonck, 2000). Clinical burned-out participants were voluntarily recruited from new enrolments of Dutch centres of expertise in burnout treatment (42%) and through the internet (58%). The burned-out and control groups were matched for gender, age and level of education in order to prevent intergroup differences that could attribute to these variables. We classified participants as "clinically burned-out" when they suffered from severe burnout complaints according to the validated cut-off points from the MBI-GS (Schaufeli et al., 2001). All participants were offered a remuneration of €25 (roughly 30 US$), to be awarded if they took part.

All burned-out participants were on sick leave; 53% were on full sick leave and 47% on partial sick leave. The average period of sick-leave was four months ($SD = 3.6$). Partial sick leave in the Netherlands occurs within the framework of a rehabilitation program: that is, when an employee is considered fit to work for only a part of the contractual working hours. Note that this sample has been used before in another different study on energy erosion and burnout (see, e.g. Sonnenschein, Sorbi, van Doornen, Schaufeli, & Maas, 2007).

Participants received an informed consent form and a one-hour instruction at home on the use of an electronic diary, which was in the form of a personal digital assistant (PDA) pocket computer. They received a telephone call two days later to discuss their first experiences of using the diary, and potential problems. Telephone support was also available during the entire recording period, which concluded with a debriefing interview and the collection of the pocket computer, and offered the remuneration. The Medical Ethics Review Committee of the Utrecht University Medical Centre approved the study.

The electronic diary study

In order to test our hypotheses, we used a technique that allows the "capturing" and assessment of flow experiences related to any kind of activity plus the time of the day – the Experience Sampling Method (ESM) (Csikszentmihalyi, Larson, & Prescott, 1977). This method allows for the repeated assessment of individuals' experiences in their natural environment (Christensen, Barrett, Bliss-Moreau, Lebo, & Kaschub, 2003; Massimini, Csikszentmihalyi, & Carli, 1987) and for the assessment of within-person fluctuations in these experiences (Bolger, Davis, & Rafaeli, 2003). In addition, this technique avoids the retrospection bias produced by questionnaires that are responded to at the end of the day or the week, because these require a remembering and cognitive integration of past experiences (Peters et al., 2000; Stone, Broderick, Shiffman, & Schwartz, 2004). In addition to accuracy and ecological validity, ESM provides the unique opportunity to acquire diurnal patterns of the flow experience. In this paper, we use the term *electronic diary* for ESM applied using a PDA.

Measurements

All variables used in this study were obtained by means of an electronic diary. The diary was programmed into a PalmOne™ PDA pocket computer with an integrated alarm and soft-touch screen, allowing for simultaneous presentation and the answering of items. The computer produced an electronic alarm (a beeping signal), which occurred randomly during the day within 2.5-hour time units to prompt participants to fill in the diary. Each participant filled in between three and seven (average five) alarm-triggered diary entries every day for two consecutive weeks. All diary entries were automatically time-stamped and the variables of the present study were assessed.

Enjoyment and absorption were assessed with single questions according to ESM premises. The items are intended to measure states rather than constructs, and they mimic an internal dialogue. They need to be concise and presented in a common language (Delespaul, 1995). Two items intended to measure flow were selected from the Utrecht Work Engagement Scale (UWES; Schaufeli et al., 2002) based on their face validity and their high factor loadings. These items are: "I enjoy what I'm doing now" (enjoyment) and "I'm engrossed in what I'm doing" (absorption). The answers were scored on a 7-point anchored Likert scale ranging from 1 = not at all to 7 = very much. Flow was thus defined as a continuous variable (cf. Csikszentmihalyi & Csikszentmihalyi, 1988; Delle Fave & Massimini, 2005) consisting of an emotional (enjoyment) and a cognitive (absorption) component that were averaged to produce an overall flow measure.

In addition to recording two flow-related experiences (i.e. enjoyment and absorption), the diary provided other information. These included the *time* of the day the electronic alarm sounded a "beep", the *day of the week*, and whether the participant was engaged in *working tasks* or *non-working tasks*. It had been explained to participants that tasks such as housework should be recorded as working tasks. (This was of particular relevance to the non-working, burned-out participants.) The study yielded a total of 5455 alarm-controlled diary entries. Participants rendered an average of 71 diary entries each, which equals a response of 81%, indicating that compliance was high in both groups. No influence of the method itself on the measurements (reactivity) was detected. Detailed information on the process of data collection in the diary study are presented elsewhere (see Sonnenschein, Sorbi, Van Doornen, & Maas, 2006).

Statistical analyses

We carried out descriptive analyses and ANOVAs using the statistical software package SPSS 15. In order to test the study hypotheses, we employed multilevel regression modelling (Hox, 2002), a method recommended for ESM data (Schwartz

& Stone, 1998) because it accounts for within-subject dependencies of data points (since diary entries are nested within days, which are nested in their turn within participants). Longitudinal data can be viewed as multilevel data, with repeated measurements nested within individuals (Hox, 2002). Within multilevel analyses, it is possible to test and compare several models starting with a null model that includes only the intercept. In the following steps, the consecutive addition of predictor variables is possible at the different levels, and the improvement of one model based on a previous one can be examined using a likelihood ratio statistic (Sonnentag, 2001). To run multilevel analyses, we employed the MlwiN 2.02 program (Rashbash, Browne, Healy, Cameron, & Charlton, 2005). In our study, data at three levels were available: at the electronic signal level (time and working tasks), at the day level (weekend or weekday), and at the person level (the healthy group or the burned-out group).

Results

Preliminary analyses

Table 1 shows the means, standard deviations and correlations between the study variables at the person level; that is to say, we aggregated diary records to obtain the individual averages (M) and the within-person variability (SD). Table 1 also shows the correlations between the variables at the same time, that is to say, at the first level, the electronic signal or time level ($N = 4017 - 5455$). As can be seen in Table 1, both components of flow substantially correlate at the person level ($r = .73$; $p < .001$) as well as at the time level ($r = .62$; $p < .001$).

Before running the multilevel analyses, we examined group differences in flow (burned-out vs. healthy) by carrying out an Analyses of Variance (ANOVA) on individual averages (M). We found significant differences between the two groups ($t = 8.70$, $p < .01$); the healthy group scored significantly higher on flow than the burned-out group. We observed the same effect for each dimension of flow separately: enjoyment ($t = 9.62$, $p < .05$) and absorption ($t = 5.68$, $p < .05$). More detailed analyses revealed that clinically burned-out participants on full sick leave exhibited no significant differences in flow compared to the clinically burned-out participants on partial sick leave ($t = .00$, $n.s.$). The same was true of each separate dimension: enjoyment ($t = .06$, $n.s.$) and absorption ($t = .05$, $n.s.$). Because no differences were observed between those on partial and full sick-leave the burned-out group was treated as a single, undifferentiated group. Thus, these preliminary analyses (to be confirmed in the multilevel analyses) led us to assert that, as we formulated in Hypothesis 1, the healthy individuals experienced more flow than those who were burned-out. Whether or not burned-out employees were on full or partial sick leave appeared to make no difference to the level of flow they experienced.

Multi-level analyses and tests of hypotheses

Before testing our Hypotheses 2 and 5, we calculated the intraclass correlation for flow in order to estimate the proportion of variance that is explained at each level (Hox, 2002). The results showed that 69% of the variance in flow was explained at

Table 1. Means, standard deviations and correlations between the study variables.

	Mean	SD	1	2	3	4	5	6	7	8
1 Time linear slope (time)	–	–	–	.99**	–.36**	.08**	.06**	.05**	.09**	–.00
2 Time quadratic slope (hour quadratic)	–	–	.99**	–	–.35**	.07**	.07**	.06**	.10**	.00
3 Working activity (0 = no; 1 = yes)	–	–	–.36**	–.35**	–	–.24**	–.30**	–.01	–.09**	.06**
4 Weekday (0 = not weekend; 1 = weekend)	–	–	.98	.88	.40	–	–.01	.05**	.07**	.01
5 Group (0 = healthy; 1 = burned-out)	–	–	.24*	.23*	–.70**	–.06	–	–.13**	–.14**	–.11**
6 Flow (Enjoyment and Absorption)	4.61	0.58	.18	.19	.14	–.19	–.29**	–	.89**	.91**
7 Enjoyment	4.74	0.60	.08	.08	.10	–.14	–.30**	.92**	–	.62**
8 Absorption	4.49	0.65	.25*	.26**	.16	–.21*	–.23*	.93**	.73**	–

Note: Below the diagonal: person-level data ($N = 100$), averaged across 15 days. Above the diagonal: electronic signal-level data ($N = 4017$–5455).
*$p < .05$; **$p < .01$.

the first level, which is at the signal (or time) level. The variance explained was 9.56% at the second level (day), and 20.64% at the third level (person), respectively. The results were evidence of the existence of three levels of analyses, as suggested by the significant proportion of variance explained by the time level, that is to say, within-person fluctuations across the 3–7 alarm-signalled occasions per day. The previous results allow us to continue with multilevel analyses.

In order to test Hypotheses 2 and 5, we tested four nested models: (1) the Null (intercept-only) Model; (2) Model 1, in which we added variables at the first level such as the time of the day, quadratic hour (or quadratic slope) and working/non-working activity; (3) Model 2, where we added the variable at the second level (type of day, i.e. weekday or weekend); and (4) Model 3, in which we added the variable at the third level (group). Table 2 presents unstandardized estimates, standard errors and t-values for all predictor variables of the four models. It also presents the deviance ($-2 \times \log$) of the four models, as well as the differences in the deviance between the nested models. A significant decrease in the deviance indicates a better fit of the model.

The analyses revealed that Model 1 showed a significant improvement in fit over the null model, so time and the hour quadratic (in terms of a curvilinear U-shape) were significantly related to flow. This means that for both groups flow exhibited a curvilinear daily pattern, whereby lower levels of flow were more frequent during working hours (10 h—16 h). In other words, the pattern found shows higher levels from 8 hours to 10 hours, lower levels from 10 hours to 16 hours, and higher levels again from 16 hours to 23 hours. Furthermore, it is notable that whether being engaged in a working activity or not had no significant effect on flow experiences.

In the next step, we compared Model 2 with Model 1. Again, this new model showed a significant improvement in fit. This indicates that including the type of day also adds to explaining flow. That is to say, weekends positively related with flow experiences, or put differently, participant's level of flow was higher during weekends than during other days of the week.

In Model 3, significant differences between the two groups were found, revealing that healthy participants scored significantly higher on flow than burned-out participants. Besides, a significant improvement was observed in comparison with the previous model (Model 2).

In conclusion, the best-fitting model was Model 3 which showed significant effects of time, weekday and group; that is, flow experiences followed a particular daily pattern (partially supporting Hypothesis 2), they occurred more at the weekend than on weekdays (not supporting Hypothesis 3), working or non-working tasks had a differential effect on flow, depending on its dimension – enjoyment or absorption (supporting Hypothesis 4), and flow levels were higher in healthy individuals than in burned-out individuals (supporting Hypothesis 1), whereas flow patterns did not differ for healthy and burned-out individuals (supporting Hypothesis 5). Hence, our results fully support Hypotheses 1 and 5, whereas Hypothesis 2 was partially supported and Hypothesis 3 was not supported. However, Table 2 shows that, at this stage, levels of flow – as assessed with the composite score – did not differ between working and non-working tasks.

Table 2. Multilevel estimates for models predicting flow experience (Enjoyment and Absorption).

	Null model			Model 1			Model 2			Model 3		
	Estimate	SE	t	Estimate	SE	t	Estimate	SE	t	Estimate	SE	t
Intercept	4.61	.06	79.43	5.16	0.25	20.92	5.13	0.25	20.80	5.36	0.26	20.89***
Time linear slope (time)				−0.08	0.03	−2.64**	−0.08	0.03	−2.70**	−0.08	0.03	−2.73**
Time quadratic slope (time2)				0.00	0.00	2.94**	0.00	0.00	3.00**	0.00	0.00	3.02**
Working activity (0 = no; 1 = yes)				−0.07	0.05	−1.44	−0.04	0.05	−0.80	−0.06	0.05	−1.12
Weekday (0 = not weekend; 1 = weekend)							0.13	0.05	2.81**	0.12	0.04	2.73**
Group (0 = healthy; 1 = burned-out)										−0.36	0.11	−3.14**
−2 × log	12102.5			12085.1			12077.2			12067.8		
Δ −2 × log				17.39**			7.90**			9.40**		
Df				3			1			1		

Note: *p <.05; **p <.01; ***p <.001.

Differentiating between flow components

In order to further investigate the negative result related to Hypothesis 3 and in order to test Hypothesis 4, a distinction was made between both components of flow. Alternative multilevel models were tested with each of the two flow components separately. Table 2 shows the results for the best-fitting model: Model 3 for enjoyment and for absorption separately. Regarding Hypothesis 3, levels of enjoyment were higher at weekends as compared to weekdays (Table 3, Model 3 enjoyment), whereas no difference for absorption was observed (Table 3, Model 3 absorption). Regarding Hypothesis 4 – as expected, enjoyment was significantly associated with non-working activities (Table 3, Model 3 enjoyment), whereas absorption was significantly associated with working activities (Table 3, Model 3 absorption). Hence, Hypotheses 4 was supported.

To summarize, the combined score of both dimensions of flow did not relate to whether the participants were engaged in working or non-working activities. The most likely explanation for this is that the two dimensions operate in different situations: it appears to be that enjoyment relates more to non-work activities, whereas absorption relates to work activities.

Discussion

The aim of this study was to explore the dynamic, daily patterns of flow using an alternative way to assess the flow experience, which has previously been measured in terms of high challenges and high skills (Csikszentmihalyi & LeFevre, 1989). In our study it was characterized by enjoyment and absorption, in both healthy and non-healthy (burned-out) individuals. The results of our study support Hypotheses 1, 4 and 5, showing that levels of flow were higher for healthy than for non-healthy individuals (Hypothesis 1); that enjoyment was related to non-working tasks whereas absorption was related to working tasks (Hypothesis 4); and (although they showed differences in actual level of flow) the daily pattern of flow did not differ between healthy and non-healthy individuals (Hypothesis 5). Hypothesis 2, which related to time of day, was partially supported since a significant quadratic slope was found, but not in the form of an *inverted* U-shape as expected, but as a genuine U-shape.

Table 3. Multilevel estimates for models predicting enjoyment and absorption separately.

Variables	Model 3: Enjoyment			Model 3: Absorption		
	Estimate	*SE*	*t*	Estimate	*SE*	*t*
Intercept	5.52	0.27	20.39***	5.18	0.30	17.15***
Time linear slope (time)	−0.09	0.03	−2.72**	−0.08	0.04	−2.21*
Time quadratic slope (time 2)	0.00	0.00	3.27**	0.00	0.00	2.22*
Working activity (0 = no; 1 = yes)	−0.03	0.05	−5.19***	0.16	0.06	2.73**
Weekday (0 = not weekend; 1 = weekend)	0.15	0.05	3.16**	0.09	0.05	1.77
Group (0 = healthy; 1 = burned-out)	−0.45	0.12	−3.86***	-0.26	0.13	−2.04*

Note: *p <.05; **p <.01; ***p <.001.
Additional findings concerning the comparison between Models Null, 1 and 2 of enjoyment and also absorption are available on request.

Hypothesis 3, relating to weekdays and weekends, was not supported because levels of flow (particularly enjoyment) were higher at weekends.

Flow patterns and their correlates

Our results suggest that flow experiences follow a diurnal curvilinear pattern. However, the linear slope was negative, and represented a flattened U-shape in which lower levels of flow are more frequent during working hours (10 h–16 h) and flow levels tend to increase at the end of the day. Two explanations may be offered for this unexpected result. Firstly, when participants leave their work they engage in leisure activities of their choosing, and specially recreation, which may be the source of the most rewarding experiences in life (Csikszentmihalyi & LeFevre, 1989). This means that our results corroborate the findings of Csikszentmihalyi and LeFevre (1989), although they used a different operationalization of flow. In other words, our results confirm the validity of our conceptualization of the flow experience as a combination of enjoyment and absorption. Secondly, we found that the effect (*t*-value) of enjoyment was larger than that of absorption (see Table 3), which means that the predictive power of the diurnal pattern was stronger for the former than for the latter. This poses some intriguing questions, such as, what is the core of the flow experience: enjoyment or absorption? Perhaps absorption plays a key role in the flow experience, at least during working activities, since estimates relating to working activity (i.e. work vs no-work) had more predictive power for absorption than for enjoyment.

On the other hand, enjoyment was better predicted at weekends than during work days and, by contrast, there was no difference in level of absorption between weekdays and weekends. Perhaps, while recovering during the weekend from the strain of the working week, individuals engage in less challenging activities which require less cognitive effort (absorption). This may be explained by the fact that people need to recuperate from the intensity of work (high cognitive effort) in low-intensity free-time activities. People therefore report more enjoyment during their leisure time (Csikszentmihalyi & LeFevre, 1989). This interpretation is also in accordance with the findings of Delle Fave and Massimini (2005), who highlighted that the core feature and most stable element of the optimal experience is the cognitive component of flow, that is absorption.

Working tasks or non-working tasks: The paradox of work

Enjoyment related positively to performing non-working tasks, whereas absorption related positively to working tasks. These results agree with previous studies that reflect that emotions such as happiness or satisfaction are higher during leisure time (Rheinberg et al., 2007) whereas concentration is more characteristic of working activities than non-working activities (Schallberger & Pfister, 2001; Schmidt et al., 2007). But why are positive emotions (or positive affect such enjoyment) frequently related to non-working tasks? Twenty years ago Csikszentmihalyi and LeFevre (1989) tried to answer this question of the so-called the "paradox of work". They argued that the fact that work activities are compulsory or obligatory, and that non-working tasks are (usually) not, may explain the negative relationship between enjoyment and work. The fact that the compulsory nature of work masks the positive experience that it engenders might be an explanation for this paradox.

However, nowadays work conditions and workers' attitudes towards work are changing, while research is also advancing on the knowledge of positive emotions at work. Therefore, we hoped that the results from the current study would shed some of light on this issue. Since we explored the functioning of enjoyment and absorption separately we emphasize that, unlike enjoyment, no affective evaluation is included in the experience of absorption. For instance, when being completely absorbed by the activity one is engaged in, it is impossible to concentrate on one's own inner feelings because all attention is focused on the activity in hand. Seen from this perspective, absorption and enjoyment seem to be relatively independent, at least at the momentary level. Although enjoyment and absorption share 36% of their variance, about twice as much of the variance is not explained. Therefore, these findings may also be viewed from hedonic and eudemonic perspectives. These assume that enjoyment is related to the former, whereas absorption is related to the latter. From a hedonic perspective, well-being is defined in terms of attaining pleasure and avoiding pain, so its core emotion is pleasure or enjoyment (Kahneman, Diener, & Schwarz, 1999). In contrast, eudemonia focuses on the full development of a person's capabilities for the growth of which engagement and absorption in challenging activities are crucial (Ryan & Deci, 2001). Thus, from a eudemonic perspective, work would be a source for development by means of challenging activities that frequently require high concentration. Hence, absorption is the hallmark of the flow experience, with enjoyment as an *a posteriori* affective evaluation (Ghani & Deshpande, 1994; Moneta & Csikszentmihalyi 1996; Trevino, & Webster, 1992). It should not be overlooked, though, that the flow experience is positive in itself – albeit *a posteriori* (Csikszentmihalyi, 1975) – and that therefore the positive affective component has to be included in the measurement of flow. So in the present study, we used the combination of absorption (cognitive) and enjoyment (affective) to assess the flow experience; the former relates positively to working tasks and the latter relates positively to non-working tasks.

Flow among healthy and burned-out individuals

Our results showed that flow *levels* in healthy individuals were significantly higher than in burned-out individuals, thus supporting Hypothesis 1. Moreover, as expected, Hypothesis 5 was also supported: that is, there were no significant differences in daily flow *patterns* between healthy and burned-out individuals. On a theoretical range of 1–7, flow scores of the healthy participants decreased from 4.9 at 6 hours to 4.7 at 15 hours, but had returned to 4.9 by the late evening (23 h –24 h). The flow scores of the burned-out participants followed a very similar pattern but were, on average, 0.3 points lower than those of the healthy participants (burned-out participants scored 4.6 in the early morning and 4.4 at 15 hours). The first finding reveals that the healthy individuals experienced higher levels of flow than burned-out individuals, which is understandable because burnout is associated with cynicism, dissatisfaction, lack of concentration and negative emotions (Le Blanc, Bakker, Peeters, van Heesch, & Schaufeli, 2001; Schaufeli & van Rhenen, 2006). However, flow patterns in the healthy and the burned-out participants were similar: even in those non-healthy participants who were on partially or fully on sick leave, the diurnal pattern was the same. Note that the non-healthy group also carried out "working" tasks, for instance, related to household work. The fact that similar daily flow patterns were found in both groups adds to the robustness of these patterns.

Strengths, weaknesses and practical implications of the study

There were two main limitations to this study. First, we did not study the concurrent validity of both conceptions of flow (the traditionally studied combination of challenges and skills vs absorption-enjoyment) by direct comparison because our main aim was to study the flow experience itself and not its prerequisites or antecedents. We considered that the inclusion of a combination of challenges and skills would complicate the electronic diary questionnaire too much and increase its duration beyond what we felt was tolerable for the participants. It would be interesting, however, to compare and test multilevel models of the flow experience with the flow antecedents, such as the combination of high challenges and high skills.

Second, even though the electronic diary is a very useful method to measure flow experiences, it also has the disadvantage that the signal-contingent strategy may interfere with the flow experience. Unlike an event-based design (in which participants complete a diary after experiencing the studied event), in the signal-contingent strategy participants should respond immediately when they hear a random signal from the PDA alarm. Consequently, we recommend that in future studies an electronic (alarm-contingent) diary is used together with an end-of-the-day diary. This combination of measures would allow the participants to register and indicate whether they had flow experiences during the day that the diary did not reflect. Another suggestion for future research is that data are collected from different kinds of job in order to compare the daily flow patterns among different occupations.

The study has also its strong points. First, conceptually speaking, the novelty of the present study lies in the study of daily flow patterns because, as far as we know, there is a lack of research exploring the diurnal pattern of flow (except Guastello et al., 1999). Second, this is the first study on flow that uses two contrasting samples (healthy vs burned-out). Finally, this study offers an alternative explanation for the "paradox of work", by differentiating between absorption and enjoyment.

This study does have potential practical implications. Understanding the daily patterns of flow experience may be useful to organizations in order to boost optimal experience of employees in the workplace. In other words, organizations may be able to take these patterns into account in order to design interventions to generate optimal experiences. Moreover, occupational health psychologists could be made aware of the relevant role that optimal experiences play in both healthy and non-healthy employees; they could then seek ways to boost flow experiences in tasks that non-healthy employees can carry out as a recovery strategy.

In short, this study allowed us to explore and find flow patterns across time, using an alternative operationalization of the phenomenon to the one that is more traditionally used. It also produced in-depth knowledge of the flow experience itself by means of an electronic diary methodology. As in previous studies on positive psychology (Clarke & Haworth, 1994; Oishi, Diener, Choi, Kim-Prieto, & Choi, 2007), we hope that the current study will encourage researchers to use the electronic diary method to investigate the flow experience, which is fascinating but at the same time tricky to study.

Acknowledgements

This research was supported by grants from the Spanish Ministry of Science and Innovation (#PSI2008-01376/PSIC) and Bancaja-UJI (#P11B2008-06 and 09I007/29). The authors wish to thank Wido Oerlemans, Despina Xanthopoulou and Cora Maas for their help and valuable comments regarding multilevel analyses.

References

Boivin, D.B., Czeisler, C.A., Dijk, D.J., Duffy, J.F., Folkard, S., Minors, D.S. et al. (1997). Complex interaction of the sleep–wake cycle and circadian phase modulates mood in healthy subjects. *Archives of General Psychiatry*, *54*, 145–152.

Bolger, N., Davis, A., & Rafaeli, E. (2003). Diary methods: Capturing life as it is lived. *Annual Review of Psychology*, *54*, 576–616.

Carli, M., Delle Fave, A., & Massimini, F. (1988). The quality of experience in the flow channels: Comparison of Italian and U.S. students. In M. Csikszentmihalyi, & I.S. Csikszentmihalyi (Eds.), *Optimal experience: Psychological studies of flow in consciousness* (pp. 288–318). New York: Cambridge University Press.

Chen, H. (2006). Flow on the net-detecting Web users' positive affects and their flow states. *Computers in Human Behavior*, *22*, 221–233.

Clark, L., Watson, D., & Leeka, J. (1989). Diurnal variation in the positive affects. *Motivation and Emotion*, *13*(3), 205–234.

Clarke, S., & Haworth, J. (1994). Flow' experience in the daily lives of sixth-form college students. *British Journal of Psychology*, *85*(4), 511–523.

Christensen, T., Barrett, L., Bliss-Moreau, E., Lebo, K., & Kaschub, C. (2003). A practical guide to experience-sampling procedures. *Journal of Happiness Studies*, *4*(1), 53–78.

Csikszentmihalyi, M. (1975). *Beyond boredom and anxiety.* San Francisco, CA: Jossey-Bass.

Csikszentmihalyi, M. (1990). *Flow: The psychology of optimal experience.* New York: Harper & Row.

Csikszentmihalyi, M., & Csikszentmihalyi, I.S. (1988). *Optimal experiences. Psychological studies of flow in consciousness.* New York: Cambridge University Press.

Csikszentmihalyi, M., Larson, R.W., & Prescott, S. (1977). The ecology of adolescent activities and experiences. *Journal of Youth Adolescence*, *6*, 281–294.

Csikszentmihalyi, M., & LeFevre, J. (1989). Optimal experience in work and leisure. *Journal of Personality and Social Psychology*, *56*, 815–822.

Delespaul, P.A.E.G. (1995). *Assessing schizophrenia in daily life: The experience sampling method.* Maastricht, The Netherlands: University Press.

Delespaul, P., Reis, H., & DeVries, M. (2004). Ecological and motivational determinants of activation: Studying compared to sports and watching TV. *Social Indicators Research*, *67*(1), 129–143.

Delle Fave, A., Bassi, M., & Massimini, F. (2003). Quality of experience and risk perception in high-altitude rock climbing. *Journal of Applied Sport Psychology*, *15*(1), 82–98.

Delle Fave, A., & Massimini, F. (2005). The investigation of optimal experience and apathy: Developmental and psychosocial implications. *European Psychologist*, *10*(4), 264–274.

Demerouti, E. (2006). Job characteristics, flow, and performance: The moderating role of conscientiousness. *Journal of Occupational Health Psychology*, *11*, 266–280.

Eisenberger, R., Jones, J.R., Stiglhamber, F., Shanock, L., & Randall, A.T. (2005). Flow experiences at work: For high need achievers alone? *Journal of Organizational Behavior*, *26*, 755–775.

Ghani, J.A., & Deshpande, S.P. (1994). Task characteristics and the experience of optimal flow in human-computer interaction. *The Journal of Psychology*, *128*, 381–391.

Guastello, S.J., Johnson, E.A., & Rieke, M.L. (1999). Nonlinear dynamics of motivational flow. *Nonlinear Dynamics, Psychology and Life Sciences*, *3*(3), 259–273.

Hedman, L., & Sharafi, P. (2004). Early use of internet-based educational resources: Effects on students' engagement modes and flow experience. *Behaviour & Information Technology*, *23*(2), 137–146.

Hox, J.J. (2002). *Multilevel analysis techniques and applications*. Mahwah, NJ: Lawrence Erlbaum Associates.

Kahneman, D., Diener, E., & Schwarz, N. (1999). *Well-being: The foundations of hedonic psychology*. New York: Russell Sage Foundation.

Koorengevel, K.M., Beersma, D.G.M, Gordjin, M.C.M., den Boer, J.A., & van den Hoofdakker, R.H. (2000). Body temperature and mood variations during forced desyncrhonization in winter depression: A preliminary report. *Biological Psychiatry*, *47*, 355–358.

Larsen, R.J., & Diener, E. (1992). Problems and promises with the circumplex model of emotion. *Review of Personality and Social Psychology*, *13*, 25–59

Larsen, R., & Kasimatis, M. (1990). Individual differences in entrainment of mood to the weekly calendar. *Journal of Personality and Social Psychology*, *58*(1), 164–171.

Le Blanc, P., Bakker, A., Peeters, M., van Heesch, N., & Schaufeli, W. (2001). Emotional job demands and burnout among oncology care providers. *Anxiety, Stress & Coping: An International Journal*, *14*(3), 243–263.

Lutz, R.J., & Guiry, M. (1994). *Intense consumption experiences: Peaks, performances, and flow*. Paper presented at the Winter Marketing Educators' Conference, St. Petersburg, FL.

Maslach, C., Schaufeli, W.B., & y Leiter, M.P. (2001). Job burnout. *Annual Review of Psychology*, *52*, 397–422.

Massimini, F., & Carli, M. (1988). The systematic assessment of flow in daily experience. In M. Csikszentmihalyi, & I. S. Csikszentmihalyi, (Eds.), *Optimal experience: Psychological studies of flow in consciousness* (pp. 288–318). New York: Cambridge University Press.

Massimini, F., Csikszentmihalyi, M., & Carli, M. (1987). The monitoring of optimal experience: A tool for psychiatric rehabilitation. *Journal of Nervous and Mental Disease*, *175*(9), 545–549.

Moneta, G.B., & Csikszentmihalyi, M. (1996). The effect of perceived challenges and skills on the quality of subjective experience. *Journal of Personality*, *64*, 275–310.

Murray, G. (2007). Diurnal mood variation in depression: A signal of disturbed circadian function? *Journal of Affective Disorders*, *102*(1), 47–53.

Murray, G., Allen, N., Trinder, J., & Burgess, H. (2002). Is weakened circadian rhythmicity a characteristic of neuroticism? *Journal of Affective Disorders*, *72*(3), 281–289.

Nakamura, J., & Csikszentmihalyi, M. (2002). The concept of flow. In C.R. Snyder & S.S. Lopez (Eds.), *Handbook of positive psychology* (pp. 89–105). Oxford, UK: Oxford University Press.

Oishi, S., Diener, E., Choi, D., Kim-Prieto, C., & Choi, I. (2007). The dynamics of daily events and well-being across cultures: When less is more. *Journal of Personality and Social Psychology*, *93*(4), 685–698.

Peters, M.L., Sorbi, M.J., Kruise, D.A., Kerssens, J.J., Verhaak, P.F.M., & Bensing, J.M. (2000). Electronic diary assessment of pain, disability and psychological adaptation in patients differing in duration of pain. *Pain*, *84*, 181–192.

Privette, G., & Bundrick, C.M. (1987). Measurement of experience: Construct and content validity of the Experience Questionnaire. *Perceptual and Motor Skills*, *65*, 315–332.

Rashbash, J., Browne, W., Healy, M., Cameron, B., & Charlton, C. (2005). *MlwiN (Version 2.02): Interactive software for multilevel analysis*. Multilevel Models Project, Institute of Education, London: University of London.

Rheinberg, F., Manig, Y., Kliegl, R., Engeser, S., & Vollmeyer, R. (2007). Flow bei der Arbeit, doch Glück in der Freizeit: Zielausrichtung, Flow und Glücksgefühle. [Flow during work but happiness during leisure time: Goals, flow-experience, and happiness]. *Zeitschrift für Arbeits und Organisationspsychologie*, *51*(3), 105–115.

Rodríguez-Sánchez, A.M., Cifre, E., Salanova, M., & Åborg, C. (2008). Technoflow among Spanish and Swedish students: A confirmatory factor multigroup analysis. *Anales de psicología*, *24*(1), 42–48.

Rossi, A.S., & Rossi, P.E. (1977). Body time and social time: Mood patterns by menstrual cycle phase and day of the week. *Social Science Research, 6*, 273–308.

Russell, J., & Carroll, J. (1999). On the bipolarity of positive and negative affect. *Psychological Bulletin, 125*(1), 3–30.

Rusting, C., & Larsen, R. (1998). Diurnal patterns of unpleasant mood: Associations with neuroticism, depression, and anxiety. *Journal of Personality, 66*(1), 85–103.

Ryan, R., & Deci, E. (2001). On happiness and human potentials: A review of research on hedonic and eudaimonic well-being. *Annual Review of Psychology, 52*, 141–166.

Salanova, M., Bakker, A., & Llorens, S. (2006). Flow at work: Evidence for a gain spiral of personal and organizational resources. *Journal of Happiness Studies, 7*(1), 1–22.

Schallberger, U., & Pfister, R. (2001). Flow-Erleben in Arbeit und Freizeit: Eine Untersuchung zum 'Paradox der Arbeit' mit der Experience Sampling Method (ESM). [Flow-experience in work and spare time: An investigation of the "Paradox of Work" using the Experience Sampling Method]. *Zeitschrift für Arbeits und Organisationspsychologie, 45*(4), 176–187.

Schaufeli, W.B., Bakker, A.B., Hoogduin, C.A.L., Schaap, C.P.D.R., & Kladler, A. (2001). On the clinical validity of the Maslach Burnout Inventory and the Burnout Measure. *Psychology and Health, 16*, 565–582.

Schaufeli, W.B., & Van Dierendonck, D. (2000). *Utrechtse Burnout Schaal: Handleiding [Utrecht Burnout Scale: Manual]*. Lisse, The Netherlands: Swets Test Publishers.

Schaufeli, W., & van Rhenen, W. (2006). Over de rol van positieve en negatieve emoties bij het welbevinden van managers: Een studie met de Job-related Affective Well-being Scale (JAWS). [The role of positive and negative emotions and the well-being of managers: A study using the Job-related Affective Wellbeing Scale. *Gedrag en Organisatie, 19*(4), 323–344.

Schaufeli, W.B., Salanova, M., González-Romá, V., & Bakker, A. (2002). The measurement of burnout and engagement: A confirmatory factor analytic approach. *Journal of Happiness Studies, 3*, 71–92.

Schaufeli, W.B., & Taris, T.W. (2005). The conceptualization and measurement of burnout: Common ground and worlds apart. *Work & Stress, 19*, 356—262.

Schmidt, C., Collette, F., Cajochen, C., & Peigneux, P. (2007). A time to think: Circadian rhythms in human cognition. *Cognitive Neuropsychology, 24*(7), 755–789.

Schwartz, J., & Stone, A. (1998). Strategies for analyzing ecological momentary assessment data. *Health Psychology, 17*(1), 6–16.

Smith, T.W. (1979). Happiness: Time trends, seasonal variations, intersurvey differences, and other mysteries. *Social Psychology Quarterly, 42*, 18–30.

Sonnenschein, M.J., Sorbi, M.J., van Doornen, L.J.P., & Maas, C.J. (2006). Feasibility of an electronic diary in clinical burnout. *International Journal of Behavioral Medicine, 13*, 315–319.

Sonnenschein, M.J., Sorbi, M.J., van Doornen, L.J.P., Schaufeli, W.B., & Maas, C.J. (2007). Electronic diary evidence on energy erosion in clinical burnout. *Journal of Occupational Health Psychology, 12*(4), 402–413.

Sonnentag, S. (2001). Work, recovery activities, and individual well-being: A diary study. *Journal of Occupational Health Psychology, 6*(3), 196–210.

Stone, A., Broderick, J., Shiffman, S., & Schwartz, J. (2004). Understanding recall of weekly pain from a momentary assessment perspective: Absolute agreement, between- and within-person consistency, and judged change in weekly pain. *Pain, 107*(1), 61–69.

Stone, A.A., Hedges, S.M., Neale, J.M., & Satin, M.S. (1985). Prospective and cross-sectional mood reports offer no evidence of a "Blue Monday" phenomenon. *Journal of Personality and Social Psychology, 49*, 129–134.

Trevino, L.K., & Webster, J. (1992). Flow in computer-mediated communication. *Communication Research, 19*, 539–573.

Effects of vacation from work on health and well-being: Lots of fun, quickly gone

Jessica de Bloom[a] Sabine A.E. Geurts[a], Toon W. Taris[a,b], Sabine Sonnentag[a,c], Carolina de Weerth[a] and Michiel A.J. Kompier[a]

[a]Department of Work and Organizational Psychology, Behavioural Science Institute, Radboud University Nijmegen, The Netherlands; [b]Department of Social and Organizational Psychology, University of Utrecht, The Netherlands; [c]Department of Work and Organizational Psychology, University of Konstanz, Germany

Although vacation from work provides a valuable opportunity for recovery, few studies have met the requirements for assessing its effects. These include taking measurements well ahead of the vacation, during the vacation and at several points in time afterwards. Our study on vacation (after-) effects focused on two related questions: (1) Do health and well-being of working individuals improve during a vacation? and (2) How long does a vacation effect last after resumption of work? In a longitudinal study covering seven weeks, 96 Dutch workers reported their health and well-being levels two weeks before a winter sports vacation, during vacation and one week, two weeks and four weeks after vacation on seven indicators. Participants' health and well-being improved during vacation on five indicators: health status, mood, tension, energy level and satisfaction. However, during the first week of work resumption, health and well-being had generally returned to pre-vacation levels. In conclusion, a winter sports vacation is associated with improvements in self-reported health and well-being among working individuals. However, these effects fade out rapidly after work resumption. We propose a framework for future vacation research and suggest investigating the role of vacation type, duration and means to prolong vacation relief.

Introduction

Research in the field of occupational health has consistently demonstrated the adverse impact of stress in the workplace on individuals' health and well-being (e.g. Belkic, Landbergis, Schnall, & Baker, 2004; Ferrie, Westerlund, Virtanen, Vahtera, & Kivimaki, 2008). This harmful effect is, in part, brought about by physiological stress responses that continue or recur during nonwork time when job stressors are no longer present (e.g. Brosschot, Van Dijk, & Thayer, 2007; Hjortskov et al., 2004). These prolonged physiological stress responses can be amplified by ruminating thoughts about past and potential future stressors (Geurts & Sonnentag, 2006) and may disturb the person's homeostatic balance ("allostasis," McEwen, 1998), that is, the balance between the sympathetic nervous system being dominant during effort expenditure (e.g. in response to stressors) and the parasympathetic nervous system being in control during rest and relaxation (e.g. recovery).

Accordingly, recovery during nonwork time plays a crucial role in protecting employees against the adverse effects of exposure to job stressors. According to Geurts and Sonnentag (2006), the essence of recovery is that

> ... the psychophysiological systems that were activated during work will return to and stabilize at a baseline level, that is, a level that appears in a situation in which no special demands are made on the individual. (p. 483)

The most influential theories on recovery, Effort-Recovery Theory (Meijman & Mulder, 1998) and Allostatic Load Theory (McEwen, 1998), share the idea that removal of demands previously put on the individual's psychobiological systems is a prerequisite for recovery to occur.

Recovery after work may occur regularly between workdays (e.g. during evening hours and during weekends) and during longer periods of off-job time such as vacations, constituting meta- and macro-recovery, respectively (Sluiter, Frings-Dresen, Meijman, & Van der Beek, 2000). Recent diary studies have revealed that workers often recover insufficiently during regular evening hours and weekends, for instance due to working overtime (Fritz & Sonnentag, 2005; Van Hooff, Geurts, Kompier, & Taris, 2007). This day-to-day incomplete recovery constitutes a high risk for serious health impairment in the long term (Van Hooff et al., 2005).

Vacation as a longer and relatively uninterrupted period of absence from work is a prime candidate for helping workers to recover more completely from work. Vacation may contribute to recovery from work through a rather passive mechanism of liberation from demands, as well as through the active engagement in valued and positively experienced free-time activities of one's own choice (e.g. family activities and hobbies).

According to Frederickson's Broaden-and-Build Theory (2001), positive emotions produce flourishing by widening people's thought-action repertoires and by building enduring resources (e.g. intellectual, physical, social and psychological). Positive emotions (e.g. joy, contentment and love) experienced during vacation may not only strengthen the social bond with partners, family members and/or friends, they may also break habitual thought patterns and lead to unusual, creative, fresh ideas to solve long-lasting (job-related) problems. Therefore, a vacation may help to build up enduring personal resources that may function as a buffer for future threats.

In the current study we therefore aim to answer two central research questions:

Question 1: Do the health and well-being of working individuals improve during a winter sports vacation (i.e. vacation effect)?

Question 2: Once a vacation effect has occurred, how long does it last after resumption of work (i.e. vacation after-effects)?

Although vacation is probably the most powerful prototypical respite occasion for working individuals, as yet surprisingly few researchers have addressed its impact on recovery from work. A recent meta-analysis of vacation research (De Bloom et al., 2009) identified only seven studies that met a set of minimum methodological requirements for studying the effects of vacation on health and well-being. The results of these studies suggest that vacation has positive, although weak effects on health and well-being, and that these effects fade out quickly after returning home. However, the evidence is still inconclusive, not only because of the small number of vacation studies but also due to suboptimal research designs often applied (De Bloom et al., 2009). We believe that an adequate study design to investigate the impact of vacation on employees' health and well-being comes down to five major criteria. In the following sections we will discuss each of them in more detail.

A proper pre-vacation baseline

A number of studies included in the meta-analysis scheduled their pre-vacation measurements shortly before participants went on vacation (De Bloom et al., 2009). However, research showed that the time before a trip can be stressful (DeFrank, Konopaske, & Ivancevich, 2000). In a similar vein, Westman (2004, 2005) stated that pre-vacation activities like planning the vacation, travelling to the vacation destination and coordinating work tasks for the period of absence may also cause pre-vacation stress. Accordingly, it is plausible that measurement occasions immediately before vacation are confounded by either "vacation preparation stress" or working to deadlines before leaving ("working ahead-stress"). But it may also be that vacationers look forward to the vacation, inducing enhanced health and well-being. In both cases, it is unreasonable to expect that levels of health and well-being in the week before vacation represent baseline levels of a regular working week. Therefore, in the current study, all comparisons to investigate vacation effects were anchored by a baseline during a regular working week, two weeks before vacation.

An on-vacation measurement occasion

A concern in some earlier vacation studies regards the absence of health and well-being measurements during the vacation period itself (for notable exceptions see Eden, 1990; Fritz & Sonnentag, 2006; Westman & Eden, 1997). In most of the earlier vacation studies, pre- and post-vacation measurements were compared, and changed levels of health and well-being were attributed to the unmeasured intervention, that is, the vacation (De Bloom et al., 2009). However, attributing a change in health and well-being to the vacation is a fallacy of the "post hoc ergo propter hoc" type ("after this, therefore because of this") because the sequential occurrence of phenomena does not mean that there is a causal relation between these phenomena (Eden, 2001).

The reason for the dominantly chosen pre-post comparisons to determine a vacation effect is presumably that obtaining data while people are on holiday is difficult (Eden, 2001). Some researchers have even described the logistics of locating people during vacation as "nightmarish" (Eden, 1990, p. 182). Furthermore, respondents might possibly not appreciate being examined during their highly valued holidays (i.e. "holy days"), and traditional research materials like paper–pencil questionnaires are hard to use in a vacation setting.

However, investigating a vacation effect by only comparing pre-vacation and post-vacation measurements is inadequate because post-vacation measurements are biased by work resumption and fade-out may already have set in. Every measurement occasion after vacation will therefore reflect an after-effect of vacation and probably underestimate the genuine vacation effect. Accordingly, the use of a pre- and post-vacation design does not allow us to disentangle vacation- and after-effects and can lead to erroneous conclusions about the effect of vacation on health and well-being. As a consequence, it is essential to obtain information about health and well-being during vacation in order to draw such conclusions. In the current study, we included two on-vacation measurement occasions and defined a "genuine" vacation effect as a significant change in health and well-being levels during vacation compared to pre-vacation baseline levels.

Multiple post-vacation measurement occasions

Insufficient attention has been paid to the fade-out process of vacation effects, once they have occurred. As a consequence, it remains largely unknown when fade-out sets in, what its exact course is and when positive after-effects of vacation have completely vanished (De Bloom et al., 2009). Vacation effects are by definition temporary, as any positive effect of vacation will fade out sooner or later, for instance, due to the renewed exposure to work demands. Because previous research suggests that vacation effects fade out rapidly (De Bloom et al., 2009), it is necessary to measure levels of health and well-being immediately after vacation.

In addition, only a few vacation studies have employed more than one post-vacation measurement occasion and, if they have done so, the time lag between the two post-vacation occasions has varied widely. In most cases, the first post-vacation occasion has been scheduled in the first week after work resumption and the second post-vacation occasion at least two weeks later (Etzion, 2003; Westman & Eden, 1997; Westman & Etzion, 2001). As a result, there has been no information available on health and well-being during the second week after vacation. To close this time gap, we collected data not only in the first week but also in the second work week after vacation.

Occasionally, previous studies have found longer lasting vacation effects (e.g. Westman & Eden, 1997). Moreover, De Lange and colleagues suggest that longitudinal studies should apply many follow-up measures that are both evenly and unevenly spaced (De Lange, Taris, Kompier, Houtman, & Bongers, 2003). Therefore, we also included a third post-vacation occasion four weeks after work resumption.

Minimalism and simple comparisons

Vacation research is complex because it necessarily involves a repeated-measures design. Comparisons between measurement occasions to investigate vacation effects and their duration should be as straightforward, logical and simple as possible. In our view, the essence of vacation research can be reduced to the vacation effect and its potential after-effects.

A vacation effect reflects the difference in health and well-being levels between the pre-vacation measurement occasion (baseline) and the on-vacation measurement occasion. A comparison of the post-vacation measurement occasions with the on-vacation measurement occasion reveals whether there may be short-term, mid-term and long-term after-effects of a vacation period. To determine when vacation effects have diminished completely (i.e. baseline levels are attained again) it makes sense to also compare post-vacation measurements with pre-vacation baseline levels.

Therefore, in our study, after-effects were investigated by comparing health and well-being levels after vacation with both on-vacation levels and pre-vacation baseline levels.

Equal and exact timing of measurement occasions for every participant

While earlier vacation studies had "... no precedent for ideal timing ..." of measurements (Westman & Eden, 1997, p. 519) and were often rather vague in reporting when exactly measurements took place, we could base the timing of our measurement occasions on earlier findings (see reasoning above) and link every occasion to an identical point in time before, during and after vacation for every single participant. Even the time of the day was kept as constant as possible.

The pre-vacation baseline levels (*Pre*) were measured two weeks before vacation. The on-vacation levels (*Inter*) were measured during vacation itself, on the second day after arrival and on the second-last day before departure. The post-vacation levels were measured during the first (*Post 1*), the second (*Post 2*) and the fourth week (*Post 3*) after returning home and resuming work. Figure 1 presents the research design employed in the study.

A *vacation effect* is present when health and well-being levels during vacation are higher than pre-vacation levels (*Pre* vs. *Inter*). The existence of a *short-term after-effect* can be detected by comparing the on-vacation measurement occasion with the first post-vacation measurement occasion (*Inter* vs. *Post 1*). In case of an improvement in health and well-being from *Pre* to *Inter* and no significant differences between *Inter* and *Post 1*, vacation effects apparently persist which is supportive of a short-term after-effect.

If post-vacation levels are lower than on-vacation levels, these post-vacation levels will be compared with pre-vacation levels to determine when baseline levels are reached again. In the case of significant differences between the pre-vacation and the first post-vacation measures (*Pre* vs. *Post 1*), vacation effects apparently endure (supportive of a short-term after-effect).

The existence of a *mid-term after-effect* will become evident by comparing the second post-vacation occasion with the on-vacation measurement occasion (*Inter* vs.

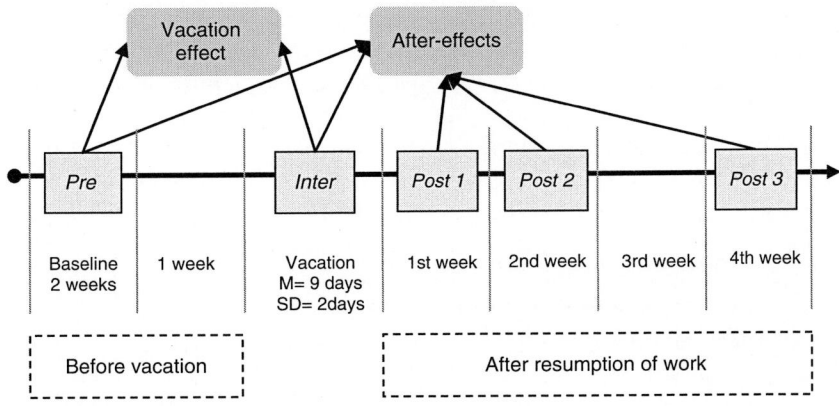

Figure 1. Research design for the current study.

Post 2) as well as with the pre-vacation levels (*Pre* vs. *Post 2*). A significant difference between the pre-vacation and the second post-vacation levels would be supportive of a mid-term after-effect.

If participants' health and well-being levels on the second post-vacation occasion are still higher than baseline levels (indicating that the vacation effect still persists), we proceed with a final set of comparisons (*Inter* vs. *Post 3* and *Pre* vs. *Post 3*) to determine if vacation has *long-term after-effects*.

Method

Data collection procedure

We carried out a longitudinal field study on winter sports vacations because this type of holiday normally covers one week and vacationers usually have no more than one or two days off before departure and after return. As a result, vacation duration and the time before and after vacation were roughly comparable for all participants. The same is true for the vacation activities that people typically engage in: winter sport activities during the day (Nordic skiing, alpine skiing, snowboarding, sledding, skating) and socializing (après-ski) in the evening. Consequently, winter sports holidays represent a type of vacation that is more uniform with respect to activities and duration than, for instance, summer vacations and therefore well suited for our research purposes.

Our study covered a time span of seven weeks around the vacation period, including the vacation itself and took place between 15 February and 15 April 2008. On all measurement occasions during working periods that is, two weeks before vacation (*Pre*), and the first (*Post 1*), second (*Post 2*) and fourth week (*Post 3*) after returning home, the participants received an e-mail with a link to a digital diary twice a week. Participants were asked to complete the diary just before bedtime on a fulltime working day. To make sure that participants would not forget to complete the digital diary in the evening, they additionally received a reminder text message (SMS) on their cell phone earlier that day.

In order to take on-vacation measures of health and well-being, the participants were provided with cell phones with international pre-paid SIM cards to take with them on holiday. They were asked to return the cell phones after returning home in a pre-stamped envelope. While on holiday, every participant was called on this cell phone and interviewed by one of the researchers on the second day after arrival and on the second-last day before departure between 5 and 7 pm (*Inter* measurement occasion).

Before the cycle of data collection started, participants received a card with an overview of their personal measurement occasions during the seven-week period. After the whole cycle of data collection, respondents were thanked for their participation, were given the opportunity to comment on the research procedure and received information about the time when the results were expected to be published in the academic literature and on our website.

To encourage participation and to reduce missing data, we announced a lottery prize among all participants: a one-week winter sports holiday for the next winter sports season. Chances of winning were higher for participants who returned all questionnaires than for participants who missed measurement occasions. In May, the winner was drawn by lot and made public. Moreover, every participant received 10 Euro as pre-paid talk credit on his or her vacation phone.

Missing data: prevention and treatment

Missing data constitute a major problem in longitudinal designs (Taris, 2000) and effective strategies to prevent and deal with missing data were applied. First of all, because we assumed that especially well-informed participants would comply with our intensive data collection procedure, we devoted much attention to instructing them on the research procedure.

Second, we scheduled two measurement occasions within each week. In order to obtain a reliable indicator of the week-level of health and well-being, the two within-week measures of a particular health and well-being indicator were averaged. This approach also served to prevent missing data in case of a single non-answered prompt during a workweek. In that case the other measurement in that week (if available) was treated as the week average.

Third, for data collection, we used electronic mail and SMS to remind the participants to fill in the questionnaires at the correct moment in time. Because we used digital diaries, we could recognize un-answered prompts immediately, and a detailed non-completion script was applied for the digital diaries as well as the telephone surveys. These strategies also reduced the amount of missing data.

Finally, in anticipation of possible technical problems with the mobile vacation phones, a sealed envelope containing a paper-and-pencil questionnaire with the interview questions was sent to the participants before departure as backup. When all attempts to reach a participant by phone failed, we sent an SMS that allowed participants to open the envelope and to fill in the questionnaire. Nine measurements during vacation were in fact paper-and-pencil questionnaires returned in a pre-stamped envelope.

In order to guarantee the reliability and comparability of the measurements, we excluded data from the digital diary (a) when participants filled in the questionnaire on nonwork days instead of on fulltime working days as requested, and (b) when participants completed the questionnaire between 6 am and 6 pm instead of just before bedtime as requested.

Considering the 10 measurements per individual, 83 respondents replied to at least eight single measurements (digital diaries and telephone interviews during vacation). Based on a maximum of 960 possible single measurements in this study (10 measurements in 96 persons), the overall completion rate was 87% (834 measurements). The combination of the 10 measurements (two measurements a week) into five occasions resulted in even more reliable week-indicators and high completion rates: 100% ($N = 96$) on *Pre*, 98% ($N = 94$) on *Inter*, 90% ($N = 86$) on *Post 1* and 96% ($N = 92$) on *Post 2* and *Post 3*. For 83 of the 96 participants data sets were complete (no missing data on any of the five occasions).

Participants

To recruit participants in the Netherlands, we distributed information via travel agencies, winter sports websites, shops for skiing-equipment, winter sports journals and newspaper ads. Additionally, we visited a winter sports fair and contacted ski-clubs (i.e. sporting clubs for skiers who jointly exercise for their next winter sports holiday).

As a result of the recruitment procedure, 176 persons indicated that they were interested in taking part in this study. After administering detailed information about the research procedure and promising confidentiality, these 176 persons received a phone call from one of the researchers. During this call, possible questions about the research scheme were answered and the participants were screened for participation prerequisites: participants (i) had to work at least 24 hours per week (18 exclusions), (ii) go on winter sports vacation for at least one week between 15 February and 15 April 2008 (22 exclusions), and (iii) enrol in the study on time (17 exclusions). Persons working extremely irregular schedules were also excluded (four exclusions). Moreover, a small number of interested persons did not want to be called during vacation (four exclusions), did not use electronic mail (five exclusions) or found the research procedure too burdensome (three exclusions). Another seven persons were excluded because they did not go on vacation after all due to sickness. All in all, of the 176 people who were initially interested, 108 met the inclusion criteria. Of those 108, 96 actually took part in the study, resulting in an 89% response rate.

The majority of this Dutch sample was male (65%), the mean age was 44 years ($SD = 10$ years) and as regards education 5% of the sample was lower (no secondary education, lower secondary or junior secondary education), 40% medium (senior general secondary and university preparation education) and 55% highly educated (higher professional and higher education). A majority of the respondents were employed (82%) while 18% were self-employed. The participants worked in a variety of sectors: 23% worked in the commercial sector, 20% were higher educated specialists (e.g. engineers, ICT-workers), 14% worked in the service sector, 12% in health care, 11% were administrative employees, 7% were craftsmen or worked in the production industry, 4% were teachers, and the remaining 9% worked in other sectors.

The participants worked in general 38 hours per week on average ($SD = 8$ hours), at least 24 contractual hours per week and the total number of weekly work hours (including overtime) varied from 24 to 60 hours. Forty-seven percent of the participants supervised other persons whereas 53% had no supervisory tasks. In terms of their personal living situation, the majority of the respondents (57%) was married and lived with at least one child, 29% were married and lived without children, 9% were unmarried and lived alone, 2% were single parents and 2% lived in their parents' house.

The mean vacation duration was nine days ($SD = 2$ days, range: 7–19 days). Vacation destinations were typical winter sports areas, with the top-three destinations being Austria (70%), France (15%) and Switzerland (6%). Most of the respondents were experienced skiers: every participant had been on a skiing vacation at least one time before, and the average number of previous skiing vacations was 22 ($SD = 15$ times).

Measures

In order to be able to give a detailed account of health and well-being, we incorporated a range of different health and well-being indicators (H&W indicators). To prevent non-response we minimized the effort required from the participants and maximized user-friendliness by reducing the number of digital diary questions as much as possible. Therefore, we employed seven single-item measures to tap the seven main indicators of health and well-being: sleep quality, health status, mood, fatigue, tension, energy level and satisfaction.

Single-item measures often have a high face validity, and participants value their directness and lack of redundant and repeated comparable items. Accordingly, multiple item measures may be validly replaced by single-item measures and still be psychometrically acceptable if the underlying constructs are sufficiently one-dimensional and unambiguous to the participants (e.g. Elo, Leppänen, & Jahkola, 2003; Van Hooff, Geurts, Taris, & Kompier, 2007).

For simplicity, we adapted response scales based on the well-known basic Dutch grade notation system ranging from 1 (extremely low/negative) to 10 (extremely high/positive) and anchored the first and the last grade. The exact wording of each single-item measure and the anchors can be found in Table 1.

Statistical approach

The data were analyzed in a 5 (Occasion: five occasions) × 7 (health and well-being: seven H&W indicators) multivariate analysis of variance (MANOVA) with repeated measures on both Occasion (the independent variable or factor) and H&W (our criterion variables). Subsequently, follow-up univariate ANOVAs were performed for each of the seven H&W indicators separately (cf. DeShon & Morris, 2003).

The *vacation effect* (Question 1) was examined by computing Fisher's Least Significant Difference (LSD) test for *Pre* versus *Inter,* presenting Cohen's *d* for paired observations (Cohen, 1988, p. 46) as an effect size. Following Cohen (1988) we distinguished among small (0 to 0.5), medium (0.5 to 0.8) and large (> 0.8) effect sizes.

In order to test if there was a *short-term after-effect* of the vacation (Question 2), we compared the on-vacation measure (*Inter*) with the first post-vacation occasion (*Post 1*). In the next step, the comparison of *Pre* versus *Post 1* told us if H&W indicators had returned to baseline levels.

For H&W indicators that did not attain baseline at *Post 1*, we examined post-hoc Fisher's LSD differences between *Inter* and *Post 2* to test if vacation effects still

Table 1.   Description of the seven single-item measures used in this study.

Health and well-being indicators	Single-item measure	A score of 1 means...	A score of 10 means...
Sleep quality	How did you sleep last night?	Very badly	Very good
Health status	How healthy did you feel today?	Very unhealthy	Very healthy
Mood	How was your mood today?	Very bad	Very good
Fatigue	How fatigued did you feel today?	Not fatigued at all	Very fatigued
Tension	How tense did you feel today?	Very calm	Very tense
Energy level	How energetic do you currently feel?	Absolutely not energetic	Very energetic
Satisfaction	How satisfied do you feel about this day?	Absolutely not satisfied	Very satisfied

persisted and a *mid-term after-effect* applied. The post-hoc Fisher's LSD test between *Pre* and *Post 2* informed us about the strength and duration of this potential mid-term after-effect.

Only in case of a mid-term after-effect, we examined the post-hoc differences between *Inter* versus *Post 3* and *Pre* versus *Post 3* to determine if there was a *long-term after-effect*.

Results

Preliminary analysis: descriptive statistics

Pearson product moment correlations were examined to determine the relationship between the seven different H&W indicators on the five measurement occasions. The full 35 by 35 table (five occasions multiplied by seven H&W indicators) is available on request from the first author.

Autocorrelations that can be interpreted as test-retest reliability coefficients ranged from .06, *ns*, for the *Pre* and *Inter* measures of sleep, to .67, $p < .001$, for the *Post 2* and *Post 3* measures of energy level. The correlations among the seven H&W indicators on the same measurement occasions ranged, for *Pre*, between $-.28$ ($p < .01$, fatigue and sleep quality) and .78 ($p < .001$, mood and satisfaction), for *Inter* between .08 (*ns*, satisfaction and energy level) and .68 ($p < .001$, mood and health status), for *Post 1* between .04 (*ns*, energy level and sleep quality) and .76 ($p < .001$, satisfaction and mood), for *Post 2* between .09 (*ns*, energy level and health status) and .82 ($p < .001$, satisfaction and mood), and for *Post 3* between $-.16$ (*ns*, tension and sleep quality) and .71 ($p < .001$, satisfaction and mood). So, the H&W indicators were interrelated, but not identical. Mean scores for the seven H&W indicators across the five measurement occasions are presented in Table 2 and Figure 2.

With regard to the on-vacation measurements of health and well-being, there were no systematic differences between reports collected by telephone interviews and the nine reports collected by paper-and-pencil questionnaires (t (85) < 1.30, $p > .05$).

Multivariate analysis

Multivariate analysis of variance revealed main effects of Occasion, $F(4,79) = 7.29$, $p < .001$, and of H&W, $F(6,77) = 140.35$, $p < .001$, as well as a significant Occasion × H&W interaction effect, $F(24,59) = 7.20$, $p < .001$. Hence, health and well-being varied significantly across the five occasions, and this across-time change was different for the various H&W indicators.

Univariate analysis

Follow-up univariate ANOVAs for the H&W indicators across the five measurement occasions revealed that the levels of six indicators varied significantly across the five occasions (Table 2). Sleep quality was the only indicator that did not show an overall occasion effect, $F(4,79) = 1.93$, *ns*, meaning that sleep quality did not differ significantly before, during and after the vacation period.

Table 2. Means and standard deviations on all five occasions and occasion effects (research question 1) and vacation effects (research question 1) and vacation after-effects (research question 2) for all health and well-being indicators (H&W indicators).

Health and well-being indicators	Means and (standard deviations) for five occasions					Occasion effect	Effect sizes (Cohen's d) for various comparisons				
							Vacation effect	Short-term after-effect		Mid-term after-effect	
	Pre	$Inter$	$Post\ 1$	$Post\ 2$	$Post\ 3$	F partial eta	Pre vs. $Inter$	$Inter$ vs. $Post\ 1$	Pre vs. $Post\ 1$	$Inter$ vs. $Post\ 2$	Pre vs. $Post\ 2$
Sleep quality	7.42 (1.05)	7.46 (1.31)	7.62 (1.00)	7.42 (1.24)	7.18 (1.26)	1.93 / 0.09	—	—	—	—	—
Health status	7.53 (1.24)	7.98 (1.26)	7.63 (1.44)	7.53 (1.12)	7.45 (1.04)	3.88** / 0.16	0.40**	−0.33*	0.08	Back to baseline at Post 1	Back to baseline at Post 1
Mood	7.28 (1.17)	8.27 (0.99)	7.41 (1.10)	7.28 (1.13)	7.31 (1.12)	15.91** / 0.45	1.01**	−0.94**	0.16	Back to baseline at Post 1	Back to baseline at Post 1
Fatigue	4.42 (1.99)	4.64 (1.99)	3.81 (1.72)	4.28 (1.62)	4.60 (1.71)	3.78** / 0.16	−0.13	0.56**	0.41**	0.22	0.10
Tension	3.43 (1.80)	2.31 (1.16)	3.25 (1.53)	3.55 (1.78)	3.71 (1.71)	21.68** / 0.52	1.01**	−0.90**	0.15	Back to baseline at Post 1	Back to baseline at Post 1
Energy level	5.90 (1.90)	6.84 (1.37)	5.96 (1.89)	5.90 (1.74)	5.51 (1.74)	9.13** / 0.32	0.65**	−0.65**	0.04	Back to baseline at Post 1	Back to baseline at Post 1
Satisfaction	7.32 (1.05)	8.14 (1.10)	7.34 (1.15)	7.25 (1.09)	7.28 (0.95)	11.43** / 0.37	0.83**	−0.84**	0.03	Back to baseline at Post 1	Back to baseline at Post 1

Note: *$p < .05$, **$p < .01$. Pre = two weeks before vacation, Inter = during vacation, Post 1 = first week of work resumption, Post 2 = second week of work resumption, Post 3 = fourth week of work resumption. Baseline = levels of health and well-being indicators two weeks before vacation (Pre).

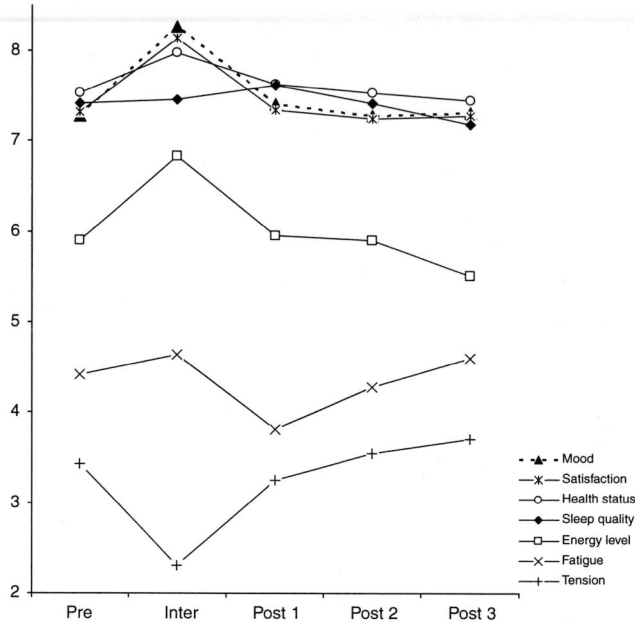

Figure 2. Line diagram of means for health and well-being indicators across the five measurement occasions.

Research question 1: Do health and well-being of working individuals improve during a winter sports vacation (i.e. vacation effect)?

To answer the first research question, we compared the pre-vacation measures of the six H&W indicators with the measures taken during vacation (*Inter*). Five out of seven indicators showed an overall occasion effect with *Pre* levels of health and well-being being significantly different from *Inter* levels ($p < .01$). During the vacation, participants felt healthier, were in a better mood, felt more energized, were more satisfied and reported lower tension than during the regular working week before they went on vacation. Effect sizes were large for satisfaction ($d = 0.83$), mood ($d = 1.01$) and tension ($d = 1.01$), medium for energy level ($d = 0.65$), and small for health status ($d = 0.40$). The level of fatigue was not significantly different during the vacation period compared to the pre-vacation baseline ($p = .74$).

Overall, self-reported health and well-being significantly improved during vacation. The mean absolute effect size d for the difference between *Pre* and *Inter* in all seven H&W indicators was 0.54, indicating a medium-sized positive vacation effect (*d*s were 0.03 for sleep, 0.40 for health status, 1.01 for mood, -0.13 for fatigue, 1.01 for tension, 0.65 for energy level, and 0.83 for satisfaction).

Research question 2: Once a vacation effect has occurred, how long does it last after work resumption (i.e. vacation after-effects)?

To test if there was a short-term after-effect, we conducted post-hoc Fisher's Least Significant Difference (LSD) tests for the difference between the on-vacation measure (*Inter*) and the first post-vacation occasion (*Post 1*). For all six H&W

indicators, there was a significant difference between *Inter* and *Post 1*. For five of the six indicators, self-reported health and well-being had declined significantly immediately after participants had returned home and resumed work. Effect sizes were small for health status ($d = -0.33$), medium for energy level ($d = -0.65$) and large for satisfaction ($d = -0.84$), tension ($d = -0.90$) and mood ($d = -0.94$). For fatigue, findings were different: levels of fatigue had decreased rather than increased directly after vacation ($d = 0.56$), indicating a positive short-term after-effect.

An inspection of the means of the H&W indicators (Table 2) already provided interesting insights: an increase from *Pre* to *Inter* was followed by an immediate decrease in health and well-being of nearly the same amount from *Inter* to *Post 1*, resulting in almost baseline levels again. The mean score for health status increased by 0.45 points during vacation and decreased by 0.35 points from *Inter* to *Post 1*. The same pattern could be observed for mood (0.99 increase during vacation, 0.86 decrease at *Post 1*), energy level (0.94 increase, 0.88 decrease), and satisfaction (0.82 increase, 0.80 decrease). Tension showed a similar pattern in the reversed direction (1.12 decrease during vacation, 0.94 increase at *Post 1*). Standardized effect sizes *d*, which enabled us to compare the rise and fall within the seven H&W indicators relative to each other, mirrored this development across time.

Post-hoc tests of the difference between *Pre* and *Post 1* were non-significant in five of the six H&W indicators, indicating that during the first week after vacation, there was a return to baseline levels for health status, mood, tension, energy level and satisfaction. The lowest levels of fatigue were found at *Post 1* and accordingly there was a significant decrease in fatigue from *Pre* to *Post 1*, resulting in a positive effect size *d* of 0.41.

Because every single H&W indicator except fatigue had reached baseline levels again at *Post 1*, we only conducted post-hoc tests for a mid-term after-effect in fatigue. As fatigue was lowest on *Post 1* and had similar levels at *Pre*, *Post 2* and *Post 3*, the differences between *Inter* versus *Post 2* and *Pre* versus *Post 2* were indeed non-significant (*p*s were .30 and .44, respectively). So, fatigue had returned to baseline levels at *Post 2*.

In conclusion, self-reported health and well-being had declined rapidly after resumption of work: five of the six H&W indicators (health status, mood, tension, energy level, satisfaction) had returned to baseline levels within the first week of work resumption (*Post 1*), meaning that vacation had no short-term, mid-term or long-term after-effect. Fatigue showed a different pattern of rise and fall, with the lowest level at *Post 1* and levels comparable to baseline at *Post 2*, suggesting a short-term after-effect.

Process evaluation

In an evaluation of the research procedure, 63% of the respondents reported to have enjoyed participating in our study and only 17% found the research procedure a little boring or time consuming. The great majority appreciated the digital diaries (94%) and 66% found the reminder SMS very useful. Only a small percentage (9%) indicated that the phone call interfered somewhat with their vacation but the great majority (65%) indicated that being called during vacation was "no problem." The majority (93%) even judged the vacation phones as a very good and creative idea.

Discussion

Vacation effect

Our study provided evidence for improvements in self-reported health and well-being during a winter sport vacation. The average effect size for the vacation effect computed across the seven health and well-being indicators was $d = 0.54$ (medium). This effect was present for five of the seven health and well-being indicators employed in this study. In particular, workers felt more satisfied and experienced more positive mood and less tension during vacation compared to a regular pre-vacation working week. In addition, although to a lesser extent, workers felt more energized and healthier during vacation than before vacation.

These findings strongly support the idea of a vacation as a powerful opportunity to recover from work demands and to benefit from positive free-time experiences. Regarding fatigue and sleep quality, participants' reports did not differ between the on-vacation and the pre-vacation occasions. The finding that mood, tension and satisfaction were more strongly affected by vacation than, for instance, health status may reflect the fact that the former aspects of health and well-being are more sensitive to changes in stressors and work demands and fluctuate more easily from day to day, than the latter.

We believe that current study has several strengths, specifically, a research design with multiple repeated measures pre-, inter- and post-vacation. We succeeded in carrying out 10 repeated measurements per individual (two measurements for each of the five occasions) during a seven-week period in a substantial group of 96 vacationers. Hereby, we applied a proper pre-vacation baseline measurement during a regular working week two weeks prior to vacation and we were able to assess the after-effects of vacation by monitoring health and well-being on three measurement occasions after vacation. Additionally, our study is one of the few studies that measured health and well-being during vacation itself. The importance of the inclusion of on-vacation measurements to determine the "genuine" vacation effect can easily be illustrated: if we had left out the on-vacation occasion, we would falsely have concluded that vacation generally had no positive effect on health and well-being.

The combination of traditional and new media gave us the opportunity to generate rich data sets in a reliable, user-friendly way and to reduce missing data and attrition drastically by acting upon the principle "the more you measure, the less the pleasure." This means, we measured frequently but in a comfortable manner by restricting the number of questions to a minimum and by designing easy-to-use instruments and resources like digital diaries, telephone surveys and SMS reminders. The process evaluation of the participants confirms that our approach was generally experienced positively.

Our findings showed that sleep quality and fatigue had not improved on-vacation compared to the pre-vacation baseline. Previous research has suggested, however, that sleep quality and stress are closely related (e.g. Akerstedt, 2006) and that sleep quality improves in times of low stress (Dahlgren, Kecklund & Akerstedt, 2005). It is possible that the potential beneficial effects of low stress and rest on sleep quality may have been outweighed by specific vacation circumstances, such as a reduced number of hours sleep, an unfamiliar sleeping environment (e.g. a different bed, different sounds, and light and temperature conditions) and changes in sleep-relevant behaviour. Regarding the latter, it is not uncommon during a winter sports vacation to drink substantial amounts of alcohol during the après ski (Meyers, Perrine, & Caetano, 1997), which might in turn lead to sleep disruption (Roehrs & Roth, 2001). It is conceivable that the beneficial effect of low stress and rest on sleep quality only occurs for those who sleep enough or consumed low amounts of alcohol before going to bed.

Hence, we tested in a number of post-hoc analyses whether the relationship between pre-vacation and during-vacation sleep quality varied as a function of the number of hours sleep and of alcohol consumption before going to sleep during vacation (i.e. the number of glasses of alcoholic beverages). These analyses revealed no main or moderator effects of sleep hours (Fs $(1, 92) < 1.26$, ns) on sleep quality. The same was true for alcohol consumption (Fs $(1, 92) < 1.20$, ns). So we concluded that neither the number of hours the participants slept, nor alcohol consumption during vacation explained why sleep quality did not improve during vacation. We cannot rule out that physical sleeping circumstances may have accounted for the absence of a vacation effect on sleep quality.

Contrary to our expectations, we found the lowest levels of fatigue immediately after vacation instead of during vacation. Strictly speaking, this effect cannot be labelled an after-effect of vacation, since levels of fatigue on vacation did not differ significantly from pre-vacation levels, indicating the absence of a vacation effect. Still, we assume that decreased levels of fatigue on post-vacation may represent a vacation after-effect: during winter sports vacation, people engage in physically demanding, uncommon activities which are presumably accompanied by feeling physically fatigued, while after work, people may feel primarily mentally fatigued.

Vacation after-effects

The results regarding vacation after-effects were less favourable for health and well-being: the five positive vacation effects had vanished within the first week of work-resumption. Fatigue constituted the only exception to this rule and was lowest immediately after vacation. Despite the absence of a vacation effect in fatigue, this finding is in line with the slower fade-out process in burnout that Westman and Eden (1997) reported and may point to positive mid-term effects regarding fatigue.

Due to the absence of on-vacation measurement occasions, most previous vacation studies defined a vacation effect as the difference between the pre-vacation and post-vacation levels in health and well-being that "sandwiched" the vacation period. Whereas the meta-analysis of De Bloom et al. (2009) revealed a small short-term after-effect, we found none in the current study. There are several possible explanations for the immediate fade-out of vacation effects that need to be discussed.

Could it be that the type of vacation is important for the duration of the vacation effects? One might argue that a winter sports vacation as a very active type of vacation may have less enduring beneficial health effects than, for example, a predominantly relaxing vacation. However, research has demonstrated that active leisure activities, in particular physical activities, improve well-being and may be even more recovering than low-effort activities like watching television (Rook & Zijlstra, 2006; Sonnentag, 2001; Sonnentag & Natter, 2004;). Accordingly, it is not very likely that the active character of a winter sports vacation explains the lack of after-effects.

Another explanation may be that a winter sports vacation normally forms an interruption of a busy period of the year. Vacationers return home and are immediately trapped in demanding daily routines and hassles like unpacking and washing clothes, work and non-work-obligations. Research on spa therapy suggests that returning home in the second half of a workweek with the weekend in prospect is more favourable for the conservation of positive effects than returning on Sunday with a full working week ahead (Strauss-Blasche, Muhry, Lehofer, Moser, & Marktl, 2004). Therefore, it would be interesting to examine in future studies whether short vacations (active or passive) scheduled at a more relaxed time of the year (e.g. during a long summer vacation) or in a different manner (e.g. one or two more days off after returning home to prevent "post-vacation stress") may have more enduring after-effects.

Third, the duration of the vacation period may constitute a major component of its effectiveness in improving health and well-being and its after-effects. Just as a lower dose of medicine may be less effective in curing a disease, a short vacation may have fewer and less profound effects on health and well-being than a long vacation period. A winter sports vacation is typically a short vacation type: most of our participants spent only nine days away from home (including two travel days) and one week away from work. As a consequence of the brief "treatment," the effects may have been weaker and more short-lived.

It may also be that in previous studies the after-effects of vacation have been overestimated. If the pre-vacation occasion is programmed immediately before vacation, it may be confounded by preparation stress for the vacation which is likely to be associated with decreased levels of health and well-being. When this pre-vacation occasion is subsequently treated as baseline, vacation after-effects would artificially increase.

Regarding the rapid fade-out process of positive vacation effects, an intriguing question may be: Why should we go on vacation at all when effects wash out so fast? However, like any other freely chosen and pleasant activity, a vacation is a period that people enjoy for its own sake; vacation makes people happy and healthy as our study unmistakably showed. A vacation is, therefore, an effective, strong and natural way to boost the well-being of employees.

Furthermore, health and well-being could deteriorate over time if people did not go on vacation, as vacation is important for long-term health and vitality, and for building up enduring personal resources and coping capacities. A study of Gump and Matthews (2000), for example, showed that not taking annual vacations was associated with a higher risk of mortality during a nine-year period. In our view, a more appropriate question regarding the temporal nature of vacation effects would correspondingly be: Is it possible to conserve positive vacation effects, and if so, which strategies can be used to slow down fade-out processes and prolong vacation relief (see also Eden, 2001)?

Limitations

The limited variation in vacation type and duration was a deliberate choice in the current study. The uniformity with respect to activities, duration and time off the job before and after vacation (maximally one or two days) enabled us to generate reliable results for short winter sports vacations. However, the question remains whether we would have found the same pattern of results for other vacation types, for other vacations durations and for other periods (seasons) of the year.

In addition, our sample of skiing enthusiasts may limit the external validity of our study. Although our sample was heterogeneous in many regards (gender, age, type of work, family background), winter sports vacationers may be above-average healthy, active and sporty. Even though we do not have theoretical reasons to assume that vacations will have less positive effects among less healthy and sporty individuals, we should be careful in generalizing our findings.

Another limitation is the use of self-reports only. However, health and well-being are by definition subjective constructs and self-reports are probably the best way to measure them (Kompier, 2005). But one may also argue that retrospective evening scores may be biased by cognitive distortions like the "rosy view bias." Mitchell, Thompson, Peterson, and Cronk (1997) found that people's post-event recollections are more positive than their evaluations of the actual experiences. Yet, we reduced such potential biases by measuring several times a week and by asking respondents to indicate their level of health and well-being on the same day.

We measured fatigue with a single-item measure because it reduced the burden put on the participants, prevented non-response and attrition and because it is a valid substitute for multiple item measures of fatigue (Van Hooff et al., 2007). In spite of that, the use of two additional single-item measures on mental and physical fatigue could have provided more in-depth information and understanding of the vacation (after-) effects of fatigue.

Finally, there may be an effect of the time of the day at which the pre- and post-vacation measures (just before going to bed) and the on-vacation measures (between 5 and 7 pm) were taken. It may be that people feel better in the early evening than just before going to bed because of feeling more tired at bedtime. Nevertheless, fatigue was highest during vacation, in the early evening, which does not point into the direction of a "before bedtime effect."

Suggestions for future vacation research

First and foremost, future vacation research could be optimized by applying research designs like the one we used with repeated measures pre-, inter- and post-vacation. Furthermore, the combination of different technically innovative instruments for data collection (digital diaries, telephone surveys) and an extensive protocol to guarantee compliance (careful recruitment, SMS reminders) may help future researchers to start measuring on vacation and to prevent attrition.

Data triangulation, for example, the combination of self-reports, ratings from the partner or fellow vacationers and performance ratings, would be a means to further improve vacation research and to generate valid and reliable results.

Some other suggestions for future vacation research regarding sleep quality (i.e. take physical sleep circumstances into account) and fatigue (i.e. distinguish mental and physical fatigue) are important and were already briefly mentioned above.

Because different types of vacation (active and passive) may have different effects on health and well-being, the impact of various vacation types on the strengths and duration of vacation effects should be investigated (see also Eden, 2001). For instance, would a relatively short relaxing vacation during the winter period have the same vacation effects and (lack of) after-effects as an active winter sports vacation? Also, the impact of similar types of vacation (e.g. physically active vacations) scheduled in different seasons of the year could be examined. Would, for instance, an active vacation in the summer (e.g. sailing or biking in the summer holidays) have the same vacation and after-effects as an active vacation in the winter?

The role of vacation duration is difficult to study because when duration varies a lot of other variables such as vacation type and activities co-vary. As a consequence, it will be impossible to attribute vacation effects and after-effects mainly to its duration. It does for example not make sense to compare vacation effects of a four-week backpacker-trip through Scandinavia with a two-week all-inclusive resort stay at Costa del Sol. Also experimentally, assigning participants to different vacation durations is practically impossible (for creative ideas like give-away paid vacations see Eden, 1990). So, the best way to study the effects of vacation duration is probably to vary vacation duration while holding vacation type as constant as possible.

Another interesting research topic is the investigation of the role of work accumulation as moderator of vacation (after-) effects. For some employees work may pile up before vacation (see also DeFrank, et al., 2000; Westman, 2004, 2005); they have to work harder in order to go on vacation and experience "working-ahead stress." On vacation, their work may accumulate even further and they may be confronted with high workload after returning home (Fritz & Sonnentag, 2006). We may call this "catch-up stress." For other employees, work may be structured in a different way and may not pile up because a colleague takes over. Accordingly, it would be interesting to include measures of "working ahead-stress" before and "catch-up stress" after vacation and study their effects on health and well-being.

A target for vacation researchers could also be the investigation of the role of vacation activities and experiences on health and well-being. Up till now, vacation remains an intervention with more or less unknown content and we do not know if vacation activities like physical activities, relaxing, household or work-related tasks have a different impact on the strength of the vacation effect or the fade-out rate (for an exception see Fritz & Sonnentag, 2006). Vacation expectations and their fulfilment, uplifts and hassles and relations with travel companions and the life partner during vacation are additional examples for possible moderators of the vacation effect which should be studied (see also Eden, 2001).

Last but not least, strategies to slow down fade-out processes and to prolong vacation relief are an important avenue for future research. Positive, frequent vacation reflection may be a prime candidate for fade-out deceleration because reflecting repeatedly and favourably on pleasant vacation experiences may reactivate positive vacation cognitions and feelings and enhance health and well-being. In an experiment on cardiovascular reactivity (Fredrickson, Mancuso, Branigan, & Tugade, 2000), positive emotions speeded up cardiovascular recovery from stress, indicating that positive emotions regulate or even undo negative emotional arousal. These findings support the assumption from Broaden-and-Build Theory (Frederickson, 2001) that positive emotions may improve individual's coping capacity to deal with stressors. So, positive emotions experienced during vacation and positive vacation reflection may protect and build resources that improve health and well-being by buffering future threats.

In conclusion, it seems that a winter sports vacation certainly improves health and well-being, but positive effects are short-lived. Future vacation studies should therefore focus on means to decelerate the fade-out process in order to prolong vacation relief. Moreover, we propose a longitudinal framework for vacation research with proper baseline-, on-vacation- and multiple post-vacation measurements (such as in the framework that we employed) to investigate the effects of different vacation types, durations, activities and experiences on health and well-being in future vacation studies.

Acknowledgements

We thank Lineke Berendsen for her help in collecting the data for this study and Pieter van Groenestijn for helping digitalizing the diaries and the preparation of the data set. Our special thanks also go to the two reviewers for their valuable, competent comments to improve our manuscript.

References

Akerstedt, T. (2006). Psychosocial stress and impaired sleep. *Scandinavian Journal of Work, Environment & Health, 32*, 493–501.

Belkic, K., Landbergis, P.A, Schnall, P.L., & Baker, D. (2004). Is job strain a major source of cardiovascular disease risk? *Scandinavian Journal of Work, Environment & Health, 30*, 85–128.

Brosschot, J.F., Van Dijk, E., & Thayer, J.F. (2007). Daily worry is related to low heart rate variability during waking and the subsequent nocturnal sleep period. *International Journal of Psychophysiology, 63*, 39–47.

Cohen, J. (1988). *Statistical power analysis for the behavioral sciences.* Hillsdale, NJ: Lawrence Erlbaum.

Dahlgren, A., Kecklund, G., & Akerstedt, T. (2005). Different levels of work-related stress and the effects on sleep, fatigue and cortisol. *Scandinavian Journal of Work, Environment & Health, 31*, 277–285.

De Bloom, J., Kompier, M., Geurts, S., De Weerth, C., Taris, T., & Sonnentag, S. (2009). Do we recover from vacation? Meta-analysis of vacation effects on health and well-being. *Journal of Occupational Health, 51*, 13–25.

DeFrank, R.S., Konopaske, R., & Ivancevich, J.M. (2000). Executive travel stress: Perils of the road warrior. *The Academy of Management Executive, 14*, 58–71.

De Lange, A.H., Taris, T.W., Kompier, M.A.J., Houtman, I.L.D., & Bongers, P.M. (2003). The very best of the millennium: Longitudinal research and the demand-control-(support) model. *Journal of Occupational Health Psychology, 8*, 282–305.

DeShon, R.P., & Morris, S.B. (2003). Modeling complex data structures: The general linear model and beyond. In S.G. Rogelberg (Ed.), *Handbook of research methods in industrial and organizational psychology* (pp. 390–411). Malden, MA: Blackwell.

Eden, D. (1990). Acute and chronic job stress, strain, and vacation relief. *Organizational Behavior and Human Decision Processes, 45*, 175–199.

Eden, D. (2001). Vacations and other respites: Studying stress on and off the job. In C. Cooper & I.T. Robertson (Eds.), *Well-being in organizations* (pp. 305–330). West Sussex, UK: John Wiley.

Elo, A., Leppänen, A., & Jahkola, A. (2003). Validity of a single-item measure of stress symptoms. *Scandinavian Journal of Work, Environment & Health, 29*, 444–451.

Etzion, D. (2003). Annual vacation: Duration of relief from job stressors and burnout. *Anxiety, Stress and Coping, 16*(2), 213–226.

Ferrie, J.E., Westerlund, H., Virtanen, M., Vahtera, J., & Kivimaki, M. (2008). Flexible labour markets and employee health. *Scandinavian Journal of Work, Environment & Health, 6*, 98–110.

Frederickson, B.L. (2001). The role of positive emotions in positive psychology: The broaden-and-build theory of positive emotions. *American Psychologist, 56*, 218–226.

Fredrickson, B.L., Mancuso, R.A., Branigan, C., & Tugade, M.M. (2000). The undoing effect of positive emotions. *Motivation and Emotion, 24*, 237–258.

Fritz, C., & Sonnentag, S. (2005). Recovery, health, and job performance: Effects of weekend experiences. *Journal of Occupational Health Psychology, 10*, 187–199.

Fritz, C., & Sonnentag, S. (2006). Recovery, well-being, and performance-related outcomes: The role of workload and vacation experiences. *Journal of Applied Psychology, 91*, 936–945.

Geurts, S.A.E., & Sonnentag, S. (2006). Recovery as an explanatory mechanism in the relation between acute stress reactions and chronic health impairment. *Scandinavian Journal of Work, Environment & Health, 32*, 482–492.

Gump, B.B., & Matthews, K.A. (2000). Are vacations good for your health? The 9-year mortality experience after the multiple risk factor intervention trial. *Psychosomatic Medicine, 62*, 608–612.

Hjortskov, N., Rissen, D., Blangsted, A.K., Fallentin, N., Lundberg, U., & Sogaard, K. (2004). The effect of mental stress on heart rate variability and blood pressure during computer work. *European Journal of Applied Physiology, 92*, 84–89.

Kompier, M. (2005). Assessing the psychosocial work environment – "subjective" versus "objective" measurement. *Scandinavian Journal of Work, Environment & Health, 31*, 405–408.

McEwen, B.S. (1998). Stress, adaptation, and disease: Allostatis and allostatic load. *Annals of the New York Academy of Science, 840*, 33–44.

Meijman, T.F., & Mulder, G. (1998). Psychological aspects of workload. In P.J.D. Drenth, H. Thierry, & C.J. de Wolff (Eds.), *Handbook of work and organizational psychology. Work psychology* (2nd ed., Vol. 2, pp. 5–33). Hove: Psychology Press.

Meyers, A.R., Perrine, M.W., & Caetano, R. (1997). Alcohol use and downhill ski injuries: A pilot study. In R.J. Johnson, C.D. Mote, Jr., & A. Ekeland (Eds.), *Skiing trauma and safety* (Vol. 11, pp. 14–22). West Conshohocken, PA: American Society for Testing and Materials.

Mitchell, T.R., Thompson, L., Peterson, E., & Cronk, R. (1997). Temporal adjustment in the evaluation of events: The "Rosy View". *Journal of Experimental Social Psychology, 33*, 421–448.

Roehrs, T., & Roth, T. (2001). Sleep, sleepiness, sleep disorders and alcohol use and abuse. *Sleep Medicine Reviews, 5*, 287–297.

Rook, J.W., & Zijlstra, F.R.H. (2006). The contribution of various types of activities to recovery. *European Journal of Work and Organizational Psychology, 15*, 218–240.

Sluiter, J.K., Frings-Dresen, M.H., Meijman, T.F., & Van der Beek, A.J. (2000). Reactivity and recovery from different types of work measured by catecholamines and cortisol: A systematic literature review. *Occupational Environmental Medicine, 57*, 289–315.

Sonnentag, S. (2001). Work, recovery activities, and individual well-being: A diary study. *Journal of Occupational Health Psychology, 6*, 196–210.

Sonnentag, S., & Natter, E. (2004). Flight attendants' daily recovery from work: Is there no place like home? *International Journal of Stress Management, 11*, 366–391.

Strauss-Blasche, G., Muhry, F., Lehofer, M., Moser, M., & Marktl, W. (2004). Time course of well-being after a three-week resort-based respite from occupational and domestic demands: Carry-over, contrast and situation effects. *Journal of Leisure Research, 36*, 293–309.

Taris, T.W. (2000). *A primer in longitudinal data analysis*. London: Sage.

Van Hooff, M.L.M., Geurts, S.A.E., Kompier, M.A.J., & Taris, T.W. (2007). Workdays, in-between workdays, and the weekend: A diary study on effort and recovery. *International Archives of Occupational and Environmental Health, 80*, 599–613.

Van Hooff, M.L.M., Geurts, S.A.E., Kompier, M.A.J., Taris, T.W., Houtman, I.L.D., & Van den Heuvel, F. (2005). Disentangling the causal relationships between work-home interference and employee health. *Scandinavian Journal of Work, Environment & Health, 31*, 15–29.

Van Hooff, M.L.M., Geurts, S.A.E., Taris, T.W., & Kompier, M.A.J. (2007). "How fatigued do you currently feel?" Convergent and discriminant validity of a single-item fatigue measure. *Journal of Occupational Health, 49*, 224–234.

Westman, M. (2004). Strategies for coping with business trips: A qualitative exploratory study. *International Journal of Stress Management, 11*(2), 167–176.

Westman, M. (2005). The impact of short business travels on the individual, the family and the organization. In A. Antonio & C. Cooper (Eds.), *Research companion to organizational health psychology* (pp. 478–491). Cheltenham, England: Edward Elgar.

Westman, M., & Eden, D. (1997). Effects of a respite from work on burnout: Vacation relief and fade-out. *Journal of Applied Psychology, 82*, 516–527.

Westman, M., & Etzion, D. (2001). The impact of vacation and job stress on burnout and absenteeism. *Psychology & Health, 16*(5), 595–606.

Work to non-work enrichment: The mediating roles of positive affect and positive work reflection

Stefanie Daniel[a] and Sabine Sonnentag[b]

[a]Department of Psychology, University of Konstanz, Konstanz, Germany; [b]Department of Psychology, School of Social Sciences, University of Mannheim, Mannheim, Germany

This longitudinal study investigates mediating variables in the enrichment process between work (work engagement) and non-work experiences (work-to-life enrichment). It is hypothesized that besides positive affect, positive work reflection during leisure time is an additional, more cognitive, pathway in the enrichment process. In total, 256 full-time employees in Germany, recruited via an online survey, answered a two-wave survey with a time lag of three months. Participants were 50% male and 50% female, and were chosen regardless of whether they had a partner or children. Analysis showed that positive affect and positive work reflection mediated the relationship between work engagement and work-to-life enrichment. These findings contribute to research on the work/non-work interface by expanding the work-family enrichment model developed by Greenhaus and Powell (2006). Our results offer practical implications for employees and organizations. Specifically, the findings show how employees and organizations can foster work-to-life enrichment by promoting work engagement, positive affect and positive work reflection. This in turn should have positive implications for both the employee and the organization.

Introduction

During the last two decades, research on the work/non-work interface has shifted its focus from investigating the negative consequences of combining multiple roles (e.g. being both an employee and a parent) to its positive consequences (Greenhaus & Powell, 2006; Grzywacz, 2000). This development is evident in Greenhaus and Powell's (2006) model of work-family enrichment. Greenhaus and Powell defined work-family enrichment as "… the extent to which experiences in one role improve the quality of life in another role." (Greenhaus & Powell, 2006, p. 73). Enrichment is a construct that captures the positive side of the work-family interface and has been shown to be conceptually independent from work-family conflict (e.g. Shockley & Singla, 2011).

Enrichment is assumed to be bi-directional (Greenhaus & Powell, 2006). In our paper, we focus on the enrichment process from work to non-work because it is more likely that organizations can directly influence what happens at the workplace than what happens in the non-work domain (Chen, Powell, & Greenhaus, 2009). Thus, investigating how experiences at work might impact on the non-work domain carries the opportunity to provide practical recommendations for organizations on how to enhance employees' work-related enrichment experiences, which in turn could affect their performance at work.

Prior research has demonstrated that work engagement is an important antecedent of work-family enrichment (Siu et al., 2010). However, still little is known about the processes by which work engagement is linked to the experience of enrichment. Our study builds on this earlier research on the relation between work engagement and enrichment and seeks to extend it. More specifically, we investigate mediating variables in the engagement-enrichment process. First of all, following the enrichment model of Greenhaus and Powell (2006), we examine positive affect as a mediator between work engagement and enrichment. Moreover, we propose that besides this affective pathway there is another indirect pathway. Ilies, Wilson, and Wagner (2009) found that the spillover from work to home is not fully mediated by positive affect, suggesting that an additional mediator operates in the spillover process. We argue that a cognitive pathway could be an additional and promising linking mechanism in the enrichment process. We propose positive work reflection (Fritz & Sonnentag, 2006) as such a cognitive pathway that links work engagement to enrichment in the non-work domain.

Until now, most of enrichment research has focused on the interface between work and family — although the enrichment concept is not limited to family in a narrow sense. We argue that employees living alone or having no children may also experience that work enriches their private lives. For example, an employee who successfully completed a large project might enjoy the evening with friends to share and celebrate this success — regardless of his or her individual family situation. Thus, we suggest extending the model of work-to-family enrichment into a model of work-to-life enrichment. This suggestion is in line with a recent call to take diversity in employees' family and non-family roles into account (Fisher, Bulger, & Smith, 2009; Keeney, Boyd, Sinha, Westring, & Ryan, 2013). Studying employees with diverse family backgrounds acknowledges that life outside work goes beyond fulfilling one's role as a family member, for instance, when taking part in volunteering activities. This approach is mindful of broader societal and demographic trends and helps to avoid unfairness perceptions of employees without children with respect to, for example, the influence of organizational policies on the work/non-work interface (Fisher et al., 2009). Additionally, studying a diverse sample improves generalizability and applicability of research findings (Fisher et al., 2009; Kreiner, 2006). Because research has shown that work-family enrichment is related to several positive job-related outcomes such as job satisfaction and job performance (e.g. Carlson, Grzywacz, & Kacmar, 2010; Carlson, Kacmar, Zivnuska, Ferguson, & Whitten, 2011) as well as to health-related variables (e.g. van Steenbergen & Ellemers, 2009), it is important to investigate enrichment and its antecedents for all employees regardless of their marital or family status.

Hence, the aim of our study is twofold. First, we examine mediating variables in the enrichment process in order to extend the still understudied knowledge about the underlying processes of enrichment. We expand the enrichment model by enclosing positive work reflection as a second pathway in addition to positive affect. Second, we extend research on the positive side of the work/non-work interplay by applying the work-family enrichment model (Greenhaus & Powell, 2006) to all employees irrespective of their marital or family status (Fisher et al., 2009). Accordingly, we will use the term work-to-life enrichment (WLE) throughout this paper. Over and above these theoretical and empirical research contributions, our findings offer practical implications for employees and organizations alike. Specifically, the results of our study point out how employees and organizations can foster work-to-life enrichment by promoting work engagement and positive work reflection.

Figure 1 shows our research model.

The relationship between work engagement and work-to-life enrichment

A core assumption of the model of enrichment is that positive experiences in one life domain foster positive experiences in another life domain (Greenhaus & Powell, 2006). Thus, it is a necessary condition for work enriching private life that an employee has positive work experiences. Work engagement as a positive, fulfilling and affective-motivational work-related state reflects such a positive work experience (Schaufeli & Bakker, 2004). Highly engaged employees have high levels of energy, are motivated to invest effort, feel enthusiastic, inspired, and proud about their work and are fully absorbed by their job (Bakker, Schaufeli, Leiter, & Taris, 2008; Xanthopoulou, Bakker, Demerouti, & Schaufeli, 2009a). High work engagement as a positive work experience is related to various positive outcomes (e.g. Bakker & Bal, 2010; Christian, Garza, & Slaughter, 2011; Xanthopoulou, Bakker, Demerouti, & Schaufeli, 2009b).

It is well documented in the literature that positive work experiences may positively influence non-work experiences (e.g. Carlson et al., 2010; Rothbard, 2001; van Steenbergen, Ellemers, & Mooijaart, 2007). Specifically, empirical research has indicated that work engagement may spill over to experiences at home (Bakker & Demerouti, 2008; Rothbard, 2001). Bakker and Demerouti (2008), for instance, described that interviewees reported a transfer of high work engagement, reflected in enthusiasm and energy at work, to non-work activities such as engaging in volunteer work. Therefore, in line with these theoretical and empirical arguments, work engagement as a positive work experience seems to be an obvious antecedent of work-to-life enrichment. Accordingly, recent

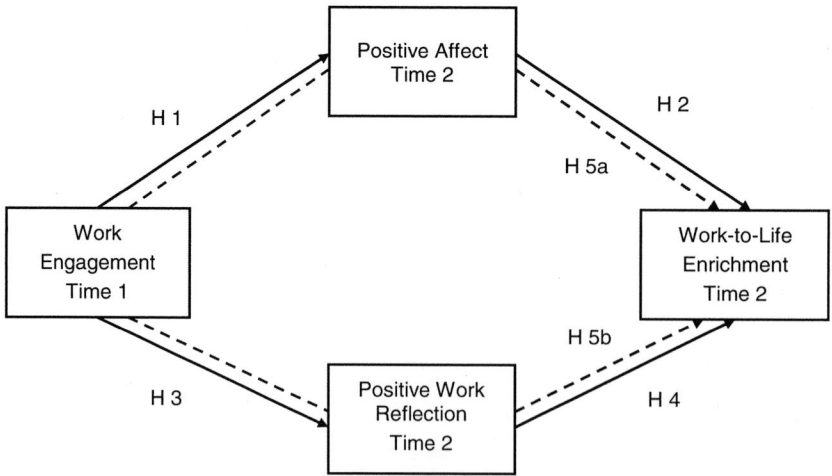

Figure 1.   Research model. Dotted lines indicate mediation pathways.

research has shown that work engagement is positively related to work-family enrichment (Siu et al., 2010).

However, it still remains to be answered how experiences of work engagement can be transferred into enrichment experiences in private life. This is an important research question, because we need to develop a better understanding of how positive experiences from one life domain transfer to another life domain (Greenhaus & Powell, 2006). We will delineate the mediating processes between work engagement and WLE in more detail below.

Linking mechanisms in the relationship between work engagement and work-to-life enrichment

The mediating role of positive affect. The model of enrichment (Greenhaus & Powell, 2006) proposes positive affect as one mediating variable through which positive experiences of one life domain are transferred to another life domain. Greenhaus and Powell (2006) argue that positive role experiences increase positive affect which in turn promotes functioning in another role.

Engaging in multiple life domains is related to an affective response (Marks, 1977; Rothbard, 2001). In this process, the quality of an experience determines if the affective response is positive or negative (Rothbard, 2001). Therefore, work engagement, defined as an affective-motivational work-related state and a positive work experience, should be positively related to positive affect (Gable, Reis, Impett, & Asher, 2004; Sonnentag, Mojza, Binnewies, & Scholl, 2008). Empirical research has indeed demonstrated a positive relationship between work engagement and positive affect (e.g. Rothbard, 2001; Sonnentag et al., 2008). Despite this empirical relationship, work engagement and positive affect have to be considered as conceptually distinct constructs. Whereas positive affect is independent from any specific context, work engagement refers to an experience that is directly linked with work (Bakker & Demerouti, 2008; Bakker et al., 2008). Moreover, work engagement is more than an affective state because it additionally comprises cognitive and motivational aspects such as being inspired by and immersed in one's work (Bakker, 2011; Bakker et al., 2008). Highly engaged employees perceive their work as meaningful and significant and are motivated to invest effort to successfully perform at work (Bakker & Bal, 2010; Siu et al., 2010). Furthermore, positive work experiences like, for example, successfully performing a work task, in turn should be related to high positive affect (Fisher & Noble, 2004; Kaplan, Bradley, Luchman, & Haynes, 2009; Siu et al., 2010) because employees feel rewarded by experiencing success (Greenhaus & Powell, 2006; Judge, Thoresen, Bono, & Patton, 2001). To sum up these theoretical arguments and empirical findings, work engagement should be positively related to positive affect.

Hypothesis 1: Work engagement at Time 1 will be positively related to positive affect at Time 2.

As mentioned above, Greenhaus and Powell (2006) suggested positive affect as a pathway between positive experiences in one life domain and the experience of enrichment in another life domain, with enhanced positive affect and role performance being the basic characteristics of this enrichment experience. To explain why positive affect plays such an important role in the enrichment process, Greenhaus and Powell (2006) built their assumptions on spillover theory (Edwards & Rothbard, 2000).

According to spillover theory, positive affect derived from one domain influences general positive affect that in turn impacts on processes in the receiving domain. These processes in the receiving domain include role performance and domain-specific affect — hence, the basic characteristics of the enrichment experience. When an employee experiences positive affect (e.g. as a consequence of high work engagement), this positive affect will not be limited to the work domain but will generalize into an overall higher level of positive affect across life domains (e.g. Eby, Maher, & Butts, 2010; Heller, Watson, & Ilies, 2004). This general positive affect energizes the employee, enabling engagement in another life domain outside work (Greenhaus & Powell, 2006; Rothbard, 2001). For instance, a high level of positive affect will help the individual to function well in the family and the wider community and to experience positive affect in these other life domains. Additionally, empirical evidence shows that positive affect broadens individuals' thought-action repertoires by activating an outward orientation and consequently helps to build new resources such as social support (Fredrickson, 2001; Fredrickson & Branigan, 2005; Fredrickson, Cohn, Coffey, Pek, & Finkel, 2008). These resources in turn can be used to enrich private life as suggested by the enrichment model (Greenhaus & Powell, 2006). Research indicated that resources such as social support are positively related to enrichment (Siu et al., 2010; Taylor, Delcampo, & Blancero, 2009). Taking together these theoretical and empirical arguments, we propose a positive relationship between positive affect and WLE:

Hypothesis 2: Positive affect at Time 2 will be positively related to work-to-life enrichment at Time 2.

The mediating role of positive work reflection. To transfer experiences from one life domain to another, employees have to integrate both life domains (Edwards & Rothbard, 2000; Kreiner, 2006). Integration of work and non-work life can be achieved via the affective pathway as delineated above (Greenhaus & Powell, 2006; Rothbard, 2001). However, as Ilies et al. (2009) stated, this affective pathway is not sufficient to explain the spillover of work experiences to non-work life. Thus, we suggest that besides positive affect as a mediator in the enrichment process, there is another indirect, more cognitive pathway, namely positive work reflection. Thinking positively about work during leisure time and thereby reliving positive work experiences while being off the job could be a pathway that links work to the non-work domain (Kreiner, 2006). Empirically, it has been shown that positive work reflection mediates the relationship between work and non-work experiences (Sonnentag & Grant, 2012).

According to Langston (1994), individuals can take advantage of positive experiences. This process is known as capitalization and is related, for example, to improved mental health and life satisfaction (Langston, 1994). Capitalization refers to the cognitive process of beneficially interpreting or appraising a positive experience and strongly draws on the basic ideas of the Cognitive Appraisal Theory (Langston, 1994; Lazarus, 1991a, 1991b). According to this theory, individuals do not just react to experiences but evaluate them as positive or negative for their own growth and/or well-being (Lazarus, 1991a). This implies that an experience influences an individual's reaction not directly but indirectly through a cognitive appraisal process. Although, originally, Cognitive Appraisal Theory refers to the appraisal of single events, the repeated experience of specific appraisals develops into a more general way of appraising a set of similar events.

In analogy to coping where repeated attempts to cope with a negative event develop into a specific coping style (Lazarus, 1993), repeated positive appraisals may accumulate into a person's general tendency to capitalize on positive events. Thus, individuals differ in the degree to which they capitalize on positive experiences.

Positive work reflection can be seen as such a capitalization approach of positively appraising work experiences (Sonnentag & Grant, 2012). It implies thinking about the positive aspects of one's job during non-work time by recollecting positive work experiences (Fritz & Sonnentag, 2006). As work engagement implies a positive and fulfilling state of mind that refers to positive cognitions about the significance of one's work (Siu et al., 2010), we assume that highly engaged employees should be more likely to think positively about their job (Gable et al., 2004). Moreover, empirical evidence suggests that positive work experiences trigger positive work reflection during leisure time (Sonnentag & Grant, 2012). Therefore, we assume that work engagement activates positive cognitions during non-work time. We propose a positive relationship between work engagement and positive work reflection during off-job hours.

Hypothesis 3: Work engagement at Time 1 will be positively related to positive work reflection during non-work time at Time 2.

We propose that positive work reflection predicts work-life enrichment. Research demonstrates that capitalization in general, and positive work reflection in particular, are positively related to improved health and well-being (Fritz & Sonnentag, 2005, 2006; Langston, 1994). Capitalization and positive work reflection, as positive appraisals of an experience, may serve as activating cognitive behaviours that help to develop new personal and social resources which in turn benefit the employee (Fritz & Sonnentag, 2006; Gable et al., 2004; Tugade & Fredrickson, 2007). More specifically, positive work reflection during non-work time should increase employees' resources, for instance, by thinking about accomplishments at work (Binnewies, Sonnentag, & Mojza, 2009). In line with the theoretical framework of the enrichment model, resources foster the enrichment process (Greenhaus & Powell, 2006; Grzywacz & Butler, 2005; Siu et al., 2010). Employees reinvest resources gained from work into another life domain, resulting in an enrichment of this domain (Greenhaus & Powell, 2006). Consequently, in line with the enrichment model, positive work reflection during non-work time should result in WLE. Thus, we hypothesize:

Hypothesis 4: Positive work reflection during non-work time at Time 2 will be positively related to work-to-life enrichment at Time 2.

Linking Hypotheses 1 and 2 and linking Hypotheses 3 and 4, we propose:

Hypothesis 5: Positive affect (H5a) and positive work reflection during non-work time (H5b) at Time 2 mediate the relationship between work engagement at Time 1 and work-to-life enrichment at Time 2.

Method

Sample and procedure

We tested our hypotheses with a two-wave longitudinal study, with a time lag of three months between the measurement points. Because it is still unknown what time frame is ideal to investigate enrichment processes, we decided on a time lag of three months for several reasons. First, a three-month time lag ensures a suitable separation of our measures to reduce the risk of a common method bias (Podsakoff, MacKenzie, Lee, &

Podsakoff, 2003). Second, a time lag of three months is not too long to seriously increase sample attrition or the influence of intervening events on the process of interest, while being long enough to provide the chance that an enrichment process between the work and non-work domain will happen.

Data were gathered by an online panel company that offers to recruit participants throughout Germany for online surveys (www.respondi.com). Survey participants could earn points that they can exchange for various rewards offered by the online panel company. We instructed the company to recruit participants who worked full time in order to make sure that all participants had approximately the same ratio of work/non-work time. In addition, we specified the sample should be half female and half male and that the final sample at Time 2 should comprise at least 200 participants.

The online panel company invited 1200 potential participants to answer the survey. At Time 1, 463 replied to the invitation (response rate 39%). Of these 463 persons, 26 were screened out by the company resulting in a sample of 437 persons who completely answered the survey at Time 1. At Time 2, all participants of the Time 1 survey got an invitation by the online panel company to take part in the second survey. A total of 281 participants answered the first and the second survey (retention rate: 64%). Due to obvious careless responses (e.g. Beach, 1989; Kurtz & Parrish, 2001) in the survey data (for instance, when participants gave the same response to all items, either at Time 1 or at Time 2) we excluded 25 participants, resulting in a final sample of 256 participants (51% women).

On average, 73% of all participants lived with a spouse or partner and 46% of the participants had at least one child. Participants' mean age was 43.6 years ($SD = 12.2$), mean work experience was 15.2 years ($SD = 12.0$), and mean job tenure was 11.4 years ($SD = 10.6$). The vast majority of our sample had a professional education (62%), 32% held a college or university degree, 3% indicated another type of professional education and 2% had no formal professional training.

We analyzed data for systematic dropout from Time 1 to Time 2 regarding work engagement, positive affect, positive work reflection and work-to-life enrichment as well as demographic variables (gender, age, having children, relationship status). Persons who remained in the sample at Time 2 did not differ from dropouts with respect to positive work reflection, work-to-life enrichment or any of the demographic variables. Differences in engagement and positive affect were marginally significant ($p < .10$). Effect sizes were small ($d = .20$ for work engagement; $d = .09$ for positive affect). Thus, we are convinced that selective attrition did not influence our study results.

Measures

All measures were assessed at Time 1 and Time 2, except for demographic data and work engagement that were assessed only at Time 1. All scales that were not yet available in a German version were translated into German by the first author and back-translated by a bilingual expert.

Work engagement. At Time 1, we measured work engagement with the nine-item version of the Utrecht Work Engagement Scale (Schaufeli, Bakker, & Salanova, 2006). The scale assesses the degree to which an individual experiences his or her work as positive and fulfilling. Items were answered on a seven-point scale ranging from 1 (*never*) to 7 (*always*). A sample item is: "At my job, I feel strong and vigorous".

Positive work reflection. We assessed positive work reflection at Time 1 and Time 2 with three items of a scale developed by Fritz and Sonnentag (2006). The scale measures how much an individual thinks about positive aspects of his or her job during leisure time. Items were answered on a five-point scale ranging from 1 (*strongly disagree*) to 5 (*strongly agree*). A sample item is: "During leisure time, I think about the good sides of my work".

Positive affect. At Time 1 and Time 2 we measured positive affect with the 10 items from the PANAS (Watson, Clark, & Tellegen, 1988). Participants were asked to indicate how they felt on a five-point scale, ranging from 1 (*not at all*) to 5 (*fully*); sample items are "interested" and "active".

Work-to-life enrichment. We assessed work-to-life enrichment at Time 1 and Time 2 with the three-item scale developed by Fisher et al. (2009). The scale measures the extent to which an individual experiences enrichment between work and private life, regardless of his or her marital or family status. Items were answered on a five-point scale ranging from 1 (*strongly disagree*) to 5 (*strongly agree*). A sample item is: "The things I do at work help me deal with personal and practical issues at home".

Construct validity

To examine whether work engagement, positive affect, positive work reflection and WLE assessed at Time 1 and positive affect, positive work reflection and WLE assessed at Time 2 represent distinct constructs, we ran Confirmatory Factor Analyses (CFA). Results of the CFA indicated that the hypothesized four-factor model at Time 1 (χ^2 = 643.664, df = 269, $p < .001$, RMSEA = .074, CFI = .922) fitted the data better than a one-factor model with all items loading on one single factor (χ^2 = 1874.410, df = 278, $p < .001$, RMSEA = .150, CFI = .666; $\Delta\chi^2$ = 1230.746, df = 9, $p < .001$), better than the best-fitting of all possible three-factor models (the best-fitting three-factor-model was a model with work engagement loading on one factor, positive affect on a second factor and positive work reflection and WLE jointly on a third factor; χ^2 = 824.771, df = 273, $p < .001$, RMSEA = .089, CFI = .884; $\Delta\chi^2$ = 181.107, df = 4, $p < .001$), and better than the best-fitting of all possible two-factor models (the best-fitting two-factor model consisted of positive affect loading on one factor and positive work reflection, work engagement and WLE jointly on a second factor; χ^2 = 1128.075, df = 276, $p < .001$, RMSEA = .110, CFI = .822; $\Delta\chi^2$ = 484.411, df = 7, $p < .001$).

The three-factor model at Time 2 (χ^2 = 205.542, df = 101, $p < .001$, RMSEA = .064, CFI = .957) fitted the data better than a one-factor model in which all items loaded on one single factor (χ^2 = 901.912, df = 106, $p < .001$, RMSEA = .172, CFI = .675; $\Delta\chi^2$ = 696.37, df = 5, $p < .001$), and the best-fitting of all possible two-factor models (the best-fitting two-factor model was a model with positive affect loading on one factor, and positive work reflection and WLE loading jointly on a second factor; $\chi^2 = 454.276$, $df = 104$, $p < .001$, RMSEA = .115, CFI = .857; $\Delta\chi^2 = 248.734$, $df = 3$, $p < .001$).

Control variables

Because we assumed that the process of work-to-life enrichment is similar to the process of work-to-family enrichment, we derived control variables from research on the work-family interface. We included gender as a control variable because research showed that gender may influence work-family experiences (Barnett & Hyde, 2001; Rothbard, 2001). Furthermore, we added relationship status and having children as control variables because the individual's family situation may influence the enrichment experiences (Chen et al., 2009). Finally, we controlled for age because this may affect the work-life interface (Carlson et al., 2011; Chen et al., 2009). Gender, having children and relationship status were measured as categorical variables. *Gender* was coded as 0 (*male*) and 1 (*female*), *having children* as 0 (*no*) and 1 (*yes*), and *relationship status* as 0 (*single*) and 1 (*having a spouse or partner*). *Age* was calculated from participants' reported year of birth.

Results

Table 1 shows means, standard deviations, zero-order correlations and Cronbach's alpha coefficients. We tested our hypotheses with a set of hierarchical regression analyses. In the first step of each analysis, we entered demographic control variables (gender, age, having children and relationship status) and Time 1 scores of the corresponding outcome variable into the equation. In the second step, we added the respective predictors as shown in the remaining tables. Finally, for testing the indirect effects (Hypothesis 5) we applied the bootstrapping approach (Preacher & Hayes, 2008). Because there is a discussion in literature if it theoretically and statistically makes sense to include control variables into hierarchical regression analyses (Spector & Brannick, 2011), we addition-ally conducted all analyses without any control variables. All results reported below remained the same. Moreover, we conducted additional analyses following a residual change score approach as described by Schaufeli, Bakker, and Van Rhenen (2009). All the results presented in this paper remained the same when using standardized residual change scores for both mediator variables.

Hypothesis 1 proposed that work engagement at Time 1 will be positively related to positive affect at Time 2. The results are shown in Table 2. In Model 1, age and positive affect at Time 1 predicted positive affect at Time 2. In Model 2, we entered work engagement at Time 1 as predictor variable. Model 2 showed a significant improvement compared to Model 1 ($\Delta R^2 = .026$, $F = 12.688$, $p < .001$). Work engagement at Time 1 was a positive predictor of positive affect at Time 2, supporting Hypothesis 1.

Hypothesis 3 stated that work engagement at Time 1 will be positively related to positive work reflection at Time 2. The results are presented in Table 3. In Model 1, only positive work reflection at Time 1 was related to positive work reflection at Time 2. In the next step, we entered work engagement at Time 1 into the model. Model 2 showed a significant improvement over Model 1 ($\Delta R^2 = .027$, $F = 9.933$, $p < .01$), with work engagement at Time 1 being positively related to positive work reflection at Time 2. This finding supports Hypothesis 3.

Table 1. Means (*M*), standard deviations (*SD*), correlations and reliabilities (Cronbach's alphas, on the diagonal) of the study variables.

	M	SD	1	2	3	4	5	6	7	8	9	10	11
1. Gender[a]	0.51	0.50											
2. Age	43.63	12.21	-.35										
3. Relationship status[b]	0.73	0.45	-.02	-.03									
4. Children[c]	0.46	0.50	-.06	.49**	.13*								
5. Positive work reflection T1[d]	2.78	0.84	.04	.05	-.04	.08	.87						
6. Positive affect T1	3.32	0.78	.01	.14*	-.06	.16*	.35**	.91					
7. Enrichment T1	2.53	0.90	-.04	.14*	-.10	.15*	.47**	.43**	.81				
8. Work engagement T1	4.36	1.27	.09	.06	-.04	.07	.47**	.61**	.52**	.96			
9. Positive work reflection T2	2.72	0.93	.02	.01	.02	.11	.54**	.29**	.32**	.40**	.89		
10. Positive affect T2	3.25	0.78	.01	.24**	.00	.14*	.23**	.66**	.37**	.53**	.24**	.90	
11. Enrichment T2	2.54	0.95	.14*	.10	-.14*	.01	.27**	.34**	.58**	.43**	.44**	.39**	.84

Notes: [a]0 = men, 1 = women; [b]0 = single, 1 = living with a spouse or partner; [c]0 = no, 1 = yes; [d]T1 = Time 1, T2 = Time 2.
*p < .05; **p < .01.

Table 2. Results of hierarchical regression analysis predicting positive affect at Time 2 from work engagement at Time 1.

	Model 1		Model 2	
	β	t	β	t
Gender[a]	.011	.226	−.006	−.130
Age	.182	3.383**	.183	3.495**
Relationship status[b]	.056	1.177	.054	1.179
Children[c]	−.059	−1.086	−.055	−1.041
Positive affect T1[d]	.649	13.753***	.524	9.060***
Work engagement T1			.204	3.562***
R^2		.463		.489
F		43.184***		39.784***
ΔR^2		.463		.026
F		43.184***		12.688***

Notes: [a]0 = men, 1 = women; [b]0 = single, 1 = living with a spouse or partner; [c]0 = no, 1 = yes; [d]T1 = Time 1.
*$p < .05$; **$p < .01$; ***$p < .001$.

Hypotheses 2 and 4 proposed that positive affect and positive work reflection at Time 2 will be positively related to WLE at Time 2. We conducted a regression analysis, entering both predictor variables simultaneously into the model. Model 1 indicated that gender, positive affect at Time 1, and WLE at Time 1 were significant predictors of WLE at Time 2 (see Table 4). In Model 2, we included positive affect and positive work reflection at Time 2 as predictor variables. Model 2 showed a significant improvement over Model 1 ($\Delta R^2 = .113$, $F = 27.433$, $p < .001$). Positive affect and positive work reflection at Time 2 were both positively related to WLE at Time 2. Thus, Hypotheses 2 and 4 are supported.

Hypothesis 5 proposed that both positive affect (H5a) and positive work reflection (H5b) at Time 2 mediated the relationship between work engagement at Time 1 and WLE

Table 3. Results of hierarchical regression analysis predicting positive work reflection at Time 2 from work engagement at Time 1.

	Model 1		Model 2	
	β	t	β	t
Gender[a]	.001	0.018	−.012	−0.226
Age	−.069	−1.130	−.074	−1.240
Relationship status[b]	.023	0.432	.027	0.514
Children[c]	.103	1.664	.098	1.617
Positive work reflection T1[d]	.538	10.140***	.451	7.661***
Work engagement T1			.186	3.152**
R^2		0.303		0.330
F		21.777***		20.451***
ΔR^2		0.303		0.027
F		21.777***		9.933**

Notes: [a]0 = men, 1 = women; [b]0 = single, 1 = living with a spouse or partner; [c]0 = no, 1 = yes; [d]T1 = Time 1.
*$p < .05$; **$p < .01$; ***$p < .001$.

Table 4.   Results of hierarchical regression analysis predicting enrichment at Time 2 from positive work reflection and positive affect at Time 2.

	Model 1		Model 2	
	β	t	β	t
Gender[a]	.111	2.211*	.110	2.413*
Age	.059	1.016	.053	0.979
Relationship status[b]	−.065	−1.267	−.089	−1.914
Children[c]	−.101	−1.714	−.120	−2.212*
Positive affect T1	.119	2.096*	−.033	−0.519
Positive work reflection T1[d]	−.019	−0.324	−.183	−3.122**
Enrichment T1	.536	8.858***	.495	8.929***
Positive affect T2			.194	3.086**
Positive work reflection T2			.356	6.466***
R^2		0.378		0.491
F		21.500***		26.383***
ΔR^2		0.378		0.113
F		21.500***		27.433***

Notes: [a]0 = men, 1 = women; [b]0 = single, 1 = living with a spouse or partner; [c]0 = no, 1 = yes; [d]T1 = Time 1, T2 = Time 2.
*$p < .05$; **$p < .01$; ***$p < .001$.

at Time 2. We tested these mediation hypotheses following the bootstrapping approach for multiple mediators as described by Preacher and Hayes (2008). We used the SPSS macro for indirect effects developed by Hayes (2008) with a bias-corrected bootstrap to calculate the 95% confidence interval, using 5000 resamples (Preacher & Hayes, 2008). We specified our model with work engagement at Time 1 as predictor, WLE at Time 2 as outcome, and both positive affect and positive work reflection at Time 2 as mediators. Additionally, we added all control variables into the analysis. The results indicated that the total indirect effect of work engagement at Time 1 on WLE at Time 2 through the proposed mediators was .18, 95% CI [.12, .26]. The specific indirect effect of work engagement at Time 1 on WLE at Time 2 through positive affect at Time 2 as a mediator was .09, 95% CI [.03, .15] and through positive work reflection at Time 2 as a mediator was .10, 95% CI [.06, .15]. Furthermore, to test if both of the mediators are equal in strength, we contrasted positive affect and positive work reflection at Time 2 within the same mediation analysis as suggested by Preacher and Hayes (2008). The results showed that the contrast effect of positive affect and positive work reflection was not significant, −.01, 95% CI [−.09, .07]. This implies that both mediators, positive affect and positive work reflection, are equal in strength, when accounting for the indirect effect of work engagement on WLE at Time 2. Taken together, the mediation analyses fully supported our Hypotheses 5a and 5b. Both positive affect and positive work reflection at Time 2 mediated the relationship between work engagement and WLE at Time 2.

Discussion

The aim of this study was to investigate mediating variables in the work-life-enrichment process. Using a longitudinal design, we tested an affective pathway as hypothesized by the enrichment model (Greenhaus & Powell, 2006). Additionally, building upon

Cognitive Appraisal Theory (Lazarus, 1991a) we proposed a cognitive pathway in the relationship between work engagement and work-to-life enrichment. Furthermore, we extended the work-family enrichment model (Greenhaus & Powell, 2006) by applying the model to all employees regardless of their relationship and family status.

The study findings support our hypotheses, thus contributing to research on the work/non-work interface in several ways. First, we broaden existing knowledge of underlying processes in the enrichment model. We found that positive work experiences (work engagement as a work-related variable) were related to positive affect, which in turn is associated with enrichment in private life (as a non-work variable). In particular, the results of our study indicate an indirect relationship between work engagement and WLE via an affective pathway. This means that highly work-engaged employees experience high positive affect, which is related to enrichment in private life. This finding supports one of the scarcely investigated core assumptions of the enrichment model, that positive affect is a mediating variable in the enrichment process (Greenhaus & Powell, 2006).

Second, we tested an additional pathway in the enrichment process between work and non-work domain experiences as suggested in earlier research (Ilies et al., 2009). We suggested that positive work reflection during leisure time may act as a cognitive mediating pathway that transfers positive experiences from work into private life. Our results show that besides positive affect there is indeed another, cognitive pathway in the relationship between work engagement and work-to-life enrichment. In particular, this finding implies that employees who are highly engaged at work are more likely to reflect positively about work during leisure time which in turn is related to increased experiences of enrichment in private life. Moreover, the contrasting analysis reveals that both mediators are equal in strength. This finding highlights the importance of a cognitive pathway in the enrichment process, in addition to an affective one. In consequence, our study offers empirical and theoretical opportunities for future research to investigate the role of cognition in the enrichment process in more detail. Summarized, results of our study suggest that highly work-engaged employees transfer their positive work experiences into private life, both by being positively activated and energized through these positive work experiences and, moreover, by thinking about the good sides of their work during leisure time — jointly resulting in an enrichment of private life.

Finally, our findings provide support for our overarching assumption that enrichment between life domains is not limited to the work-*family* interface. We found that high work engagement is related to enrichment in private life in general. These results suggest that enrichment can be an experience of all employees regardless of their relationship or family status. Provided that the consequences of work-life enrichment is similar to work-family enrichment, this is an important finding because work-family enrichment has been shown to be related to several positive consequences such as improved well-being, physical health, job performance (e.g. Carlson et al., 2011; Rantanen, Kinnunen, Mauno, & Tement, 2013; van Steenbergen & Ellemers, 2009) and job satisfaction (Shockley & Singla, 2011). Because these variables are important criteria within the individual as well as the organizational context, future research should investigate the relationship between WLE and crucial organizational and individual outcomes.

To summarize, our study contributes theoretically and empirically to the understanding of the enrichment process in the work/non-work interplay. In particular, it sheds light on mediating variables underlying the enrichment process, thus expanding existing research and theory on the work/non-work interface (e.g. Fisher et al., 2009; Greenhaus & Powell, 2006; Siu et al., 2010). First of all, our results support the core assumption of the enrichment model that positive affect is an essential mediator in the enrichment process. Secondly, our study is in line with the proposition derived from Cognitive Appraisal Theory (Lazarus, 1991a) that in addition to the affective there is a cognitive pathway, namely positive work reflection that links positive work experiences to enrichment in private life. Additionally, we showed that the work-family enrichment model developed by Greenhaus and Powell (2006) can be extended and applied to all employees — regardless of their relationship or family status.

Limitations and future research

Despite these theoretical and empirical contributions, our study has some limitations. First of all, we used self-report measures for all constructs, raising questions about common-method bias (Podsakoff et al., 2003). However, due to the longitudinal study design we could temporally separate the measurement of predictor and outcome variables, which can partially rule out self-source bias. Moreover, confirmatory factor analyses demonstrated that our study variables are independent constructs at both measurement points. Nevertheless, future research might want to replicate our findings by using ratings from other sources such as friends or relatives. Additionally, it has to be noted that mediators and outcome variables were measured simultaneously, which may increase spurious relations between the variables. Therefore, researchers might want to implement a three-wave study design, so that mediators and outcome variables can be assessed at distinct points in time, in order to reduce the likelihood of inflated associations.

A further limitation in our study might be the relatively low response rate (38.6%). Low response rates are a well-known problem in online panel surveys and might be caused, for example, by the fact that invitation mails are perceived as junk mails or that the database of potential participants is not well maintained (Evans & Mathur, 2006). However, online panel surveys also offer several advantages, such as providing a controlled sample (Evans & Mathur, 2006). Because we intended in our study to investigate a very specific sample (gender-balanced, working full-time, diverse occupations), the advantages of the online panel survey outweigh the disadvantage of a low response rate.

The findings of our study suggest a causal relationship between predictor, mediator and outcome variables. Yet, although predictor and outcome variables were collected at different measurement points in order to rule out some alternative explanations, our research design does not allow for clear causal inferences. Therefore, future research might conduct an experimental study and manipulate, for example, positive work reflection and positive affect to strengthen the findings of our field study.

Finally, as mentioned above, work-to-family enrichment is related to several favourable outcomes (e.g. Carlson et al., 2011). Therefore, future research should investigate the relationship between enrichment of private life and important outcomes such as physical and mental health and job performance to confirm the assumption that consequences of WLE are comparable to those of work-to-family enrichment.

Theoretical and practical implications

Based on Cognitive Appraisal Theory (Lazarus, 1991a), this study contributes to research on mediating variables in the enrichment process between the work and non-work domains. Our results demonstrate that besides positive affect there is a cognitive pathway linking positive work experiences to positive experiences in private life. This finding suggests that the model of enrichment (Greenhaus & Powell, 2006) should be expanded by an additional, namely cognitive pathway. As the present study is the first to investigate a cognitive pathway in the enrichment process, future research should replicate our findings. Furthermore, the results of our study might encourage the examination of additional facets of cognitive appraisal in the work/non-work interface (van Steenbergen, Ellemers, Haslam, & Urlings, 2008). Additionally, it might be an interesting research question to investigate whether there are any moderating variables that influence the mediating mechanisms, for example, employees' strategies to manage boundaries between work and non-work (Ilies et al., 2009).

Cognitive Appraisal Theory proposes that although appraisal and emotion are distinct constructs they may depend on each other (Lazarus, 1991a). Thus, as our study design does not allow the testing of causal relationships between the mediators, future research might examine this relationship by using, for example, a diary design with multiple measurement points. Additionally, the Cognitive Appraisal Theory (Lazarus, 1991a, 1991b) assumes that cognitive appraisals might depend on specific situations that vary across different situations and over time. Because our study design took up a longitudinal perspective, we were not able to examine variations across different situations and time lags. Thus, future researchers might want to study these different perspectives on cognitive appraisals in the enrichment process by combining a longitudinal — as an inter-individual approach — with an approach that focuses on intra-individual changes over time and across situations, for example, by means of a diary study or event sampling method.

Besides these theoretical implications, the results of our study offer practical implications for both organizations and individual employees. If one assumes that work-to-*family* enrichment and work-to-*life* enrichment are similar in their consequences, organizations should foster WLE and thus improve employee's job satisfaction and, in consequence, their job performance. Therefore, as work engagement is an antecedent of WLE, organizations and supervisors should enhance employee's work engagement. A growing body of research shows that job resources are positively related to work engagement (Christian et al., 2011; Crawford, LePine, & Rich, 2010; Demerouti, Bakker, Nachreiner, & Schaufeli, 2001). In consequence, organizations should provide job resources in order to enhance employees' work engagement and, in turn, WLE. Additionally, employees themselves could actively take advantage and benefit from positive work experiences.

The results of our study indicated that positive work reflection is a mediator in the relationship between work engagement and WLE. This implies that employees do not simply react emotionally to positive experiences but actively reflect on them (Lazarus, 1991a) which in turn results in a positive outcome, such as the enrichment of private life. As individuals may actively influence their thoughts (Piotrkowski, 1979), this opens the chance for employees to increase their own WLE by integrating the positive aspects of their job into their private life by, for example, thinking about their accomplishments and other positive experiences at work. For that purpose, employees themselves may trigger positive work reflection by, for example, sharing positive work experiences with important others (Gable et al., 2004). In addition, employees can foster positive work reflection by implementing cognitive routines during leisure time and thinking about the positive sides of their work.

Overall, our study indicates that both affective and cognitive processes are important for work-to-life enrichment, which in turn might benefit both the employee and the employer.

References

Bakker, A. B. (2011). An evidence-based model of work engagement. *Current Directions in Psychological Science, 20*, 265–269.

Bakker, A. B., & Bal, P. M. (2010). Weekly work engagement and performance: A study among starting teachers. *Journal of Occupational and Organizational Psychology, 83*(1), 189–206.

Bakker, A. B., & Demerouti, E. (2008). Towards a model of work engagement. *The Career Development International, 13*, 209–223.

Bakker, A. B., Schaufeli, W. B., Leiter, M. P., & Taris, T. W. (2008). Work engagement: An emerging concept in occupational health psychology. *Work & Stress, 22*, 187–200.

Barnett, R. C., & Hyde, J. S. (2001). Women, men, work, and family. *American Psychologist, 56*, 781–796.

Beach, D. A. (1989). Identifying the random responder. *The Journal of Psychology: Interdisciplinary and Applied, 123*(1), 101–103.

Binnewies, C., Sonnentag, S., & Mojza, E. J. (2009). Feeling recovered and thinking about the good sides of one's work. *Journal of Occupational Health Psychology, 14*, 243–256.

Carlson, D. S., Grzywacz, J. G., & Kacmar, K. M. (2010). The relationship of schedule flexibility and outcomes via the work-family interface. *Journal of Managerial Psychology, 25*, 330–355.

Carlson, D. S., Kacmar, K. M., Zivnuska, S., Ferguson, M., & Whitten, D. (2011). Work-family enrichment and job performance: A constructive replication of affective events theory. *Journal of Occupational Health Psychology, 16*, 297–312.

Chen, Z., Powell, G. N., & Greenhaus, J. H. (2009). Work-to-family conflict, positive spillover, and boundary management: A person-environment fit approach. *Journal of Vocational Behavior, 74*(1), 82–93.

Christian, M. S., Garza, A. S., & Slaughter, J. E. (2011). Work engagement: A quantitative review and test of its relations with task and contextual performance. *Personnel Psychology, 64*(1), 89–136.

Crawford, E. R., LePine, J. A., & Rich, B. L. (2010). Linking job demands and resources to employee engagement and burnout: A theoretical extension and meta-analytic test. *Journal of Applied Psychology, 95*, 834–848.

Demerouti, E., Bakker, A. B., Nachreiner, F., & Schaufeli, W. B. (2001). The job demands-resources model of burnout. *Journal of Applied Psychology, 86*, 499–512.

Eby, L. T., Maher, C. P., & Butts, M. M. (2010). The intersection of work and family life: The role of affect. *Annual Review of Psychology, 61*, 599–622.

Edwards, J. R., & Rothbard, N. P. (2000). Mechanisms linking work and family: Clarifying the relationship between work and family constructs. *Academy of Management Review, 25*, 178–199.

Evans, J. R., & Mathur, A. (2006). The value of online surveys. *Internet Research, 15*, 195–219.

Fisher, G. G., Bulger, C. A., & Smith, C. S. (2009). Beyond work and family: A measure of work/ nonwork interference and enhancement. *Journal of Occupational Health Psychology, 14*, 441–456.

Fisher, C. D., & Noble, C. S. (2004). A within-person examination of correlates of performance and emotions while working. *Human Performance, 17*, 145–168.

Fredrickson, B. L. (2001). The role of positive emotions in positive psychology: The broaden-and-build theory of positive emotions. *American Psychologist, 56*, 218–226.

Fredrickson, B. L., & Branigan, C. (2005). Positive emotions broaden the scope of attention and thought-action repertoires. *Cognition and Emotion, 19*, 313–332.

Fredrickson, B. L., Cohn, M. A., Coffey, K. A., Pek, J., & Finkel, S. M. (2008). Open hearts build lives: Positive emotions, induced through loving-kindness meditation, build consequential personal resources. *Journal of Personality and Social Psychology, 95*, 1045–1062.

Fritz, C., & Sonnentag, S. (2005). Recovery, health, and job performance: Effects of weekend experiences. *Journal of Occupational Health Psychology, 10*, 187–199.

Fritz, C., & Sonnentag, S. (2006). Recovery, well-being, and performance-related outcomes: The role of workload and vacation experiences. *Journal of Applied Psychology, 91*, 936–945.

Gable, S. L., Reis, H. T., Impett, E. A., & Asher, E. R. (2004). What do you do when things go right? The intrapersonal and interpersonal benefits of sharing positive events. *Journal of Personality and Social Psychology, 87*, 228–245.

Greenhaus, J. H., & Powell, G. N. (2006). When work and family are allies: A theory of work-family enrichment. *Academy of Management Review, 31*(1), 72–92.

Grzywacz, J. G. (2000). Work-family spillover and health during midlife: Is managing conflict everything? *American Journal of Health Promotion, 14*, 236–243.

Grzywacz, J. G., & Butler, A. B. (2005). The impact of job characteristics on work-to-family facilitation: Testing a theory and distinguishing a construct. *Journal of Occupational Health Psychology, 10*(2), 97–109.

Hayes, A. F. (2008, 2011). *SPSS macro for estimating total indirect and specific indirect effects in multiple mediator models.* Retrieved from http://www.afhayes.com/spss-sas-and-mplus-macros-and-code.html#indirect

Heller, D., Watson, D., & Ilies, R. (2004). The role of person versus situation in life satisfaction: A critical examination. *Psychological Bulletin, 130*, 574–600.

Ilies, R., Wilson, K. S., & Wagner, D. T. (2009). The spillover of daily job satisfaction onto employees' family lives: The facilitating role of work-family integration. *Academy of Management Journal, 52*(1), 87–102.

Judge, T. A., Thoresen, C. J., Bono, J. E., & Patton, G. K. (2001). The job satisfaction–job performance relationship: A qualitative and quantitative review. *Psychological Bulletin, 127*, 376–407.

Kaplan, S., Bradley, J. C., Luchman, J. N., & Haynes, D. (2009). On the role of positive and negative affectivity in job performance: A meta-analytic investigation. *Journal of Applied Psychology, 94*, 162–176.

Keeney, J., Boyd, E. M., Sinha, R., Westring, A. F., & Ryan, A. M. (2013). From "work–family" to "work–life": Broadening our conceptualization and measurement. *Journal of Vocational Behavior, 82*, 221–237.

Kreiner, G. E. (2006). Consequences of work-home segmentation or integration: A person-environment fit perspective. *Journal of Organizational Behavior, 27*, 485–507.

Kurtz, J. E., & Parrish, C. L. (2001). Semantic response consistency and protocol validity in structured personality assessment: The case of the NEO-PI-R. *Journal of Personality Assessment, 76*, 315–332.

Langston, C. A. (1994). Capitalizing on and coping with daily-life events: Expressive responses to positive events. *Journal of Personality and Social Psychology, 67*, 1112–1125.

Lazarus, R. S. (1991a). Cognition and motivation in emotion. *American Psychologist, 46*, 352–367.

Lazarus, R. S. (1991b). Progress on a cognitive-motivational-relational theory of emotion. *American Psychologist, 46*, 819–834.

Lazarus, R. S. (1993). Coping theory and research: Past, present, and future. *Psychosomatic Medicine, 55*, 234–247.

Marks, S. R. (1977). Multiple roles and role strain: Some notes on human energy, time and commitment. *American Sociological Review, 42*, 921–936.

Piotrkowski, C. S. (1979). *Work and the family system.* New York, NY: Free Press.

Podsakoff, P. M., MacKenzie, S. B., Lee, J.-Y., & Podsakoff, N. P. (2003). Common method biases in behavioral research: A critical review of the literature and recommended remedies. *Journal of Applied Psychology, 88*, 879–903.

Preacher, K. J., & Hayes, A. F. (2008). Asymptotic and resampling strategies for assessing and comparing indirect effects in multiple mediator models. *Behavior Research Methods, 40*, 879–891.

Rantanen, J., Kinnunen, U., Mauno, S., & Tement, S. (2013). Patterns of conflict and enrichment in work-family balance: A three-dimensional typology. *Work & Stress, 27*, 141–163.

Rothbard, N. P. (2001). Enriching or depleting? The dynamics of engagement in work and family roles. *Administrative Science Quarterly, 46*, 655–684.

Schaufeli, W. B., & Bakker, A. B. (2004). Job demands, job resources, and their relationship with burnout and engagement: A multi-sample study. *Journal of Organizational Behavior, 25*, 293–315.

Schaufeli, W. B., Bakker, A. B., & Salanova, M. (2006). The measurement of work engagement with a short questionnaire: A cross-national study. *Educational and Psychological Measurement, 66*, 701–716.

Schaufeli, W. B., Bakker, A. B., & Van Rhenen, W. (2009). How changes in job demands and resources predict burnout, work engagement and sickness absenteeism. *Journal of Organizational Behavior, 30,* 893–917.

Shockley, K. M., & Singla, N. (2011). Reconsidering work-family interactions and satisfaction: A meta-analysis. *Journal of Management, 37,* 861–886.

Siu, O.-l., Lu, J.-f., Brough, P., Lu, C.-q., Bakker, A. B., Kalliath, T., … Shi, K. (2010). Role resources and work family enrichment: The role of work engagement. *Journal of Vocational Behavior, 77,* 470–480.

Sonnentag, S., & Grant, A. M. (2012). Doing good at work feels good at home, but not right away: When and why perceived prosocial impact predicts positive affect. *Personnel Psychology, 65,* 495–530.

Sonnentag, S., Mojza, E. J., Binnewies, C., & Scholl, A. (2008). Being engaged at work and detached at home: A week-level study on work engagement, psychological detachment, and affect. *Work & Stress, 22,* 257–276.

Spector, P. E., & Brannick, M. T. (2011). Methodological urban legends: The misuse of statistical control variables. *Organizational Research Methods, 14,* 287–305.

Taylor, B. L., Delcampo, R. G., & Blancero, D. M. (2009). Work-family conflict/facilitation and the role of workplace supports for U.S. Hispanic professionals. *Journal of Organizational Behavior, 30,* 643–664.

Tugade, M. M., & Fredrickson, B. L. (2007). Regulation of positive emotions: Emotion regulation strategies that promote resilience. *Journal of Happiness Studies, 8,* 311–333.

van Steenbergen, E. F., & Ellemers, N. (2009). Is managing the work-family interface worthwhile? Benefits for employee health and performance. *Journal of Organizational Behavior, 30,* 617–642.

van Steenbergen, E. F., Ellemers, N., Haslam, S. A., & Urlings, F. (2008). There is nothing either good or bad but thinking makes it so: Informational support and cognitive appraisal of the work-family interface. *Journal of Occupational and Organizational Psychology, 81,* 349–367.

van Steenbergen, E. F., Ellemers, N., & Mooijaart, A. (2007). How work and family can facilitate each other: Distinct types of work-family facilitation and outcomes for women and men. *Journal of Occupational Health Psychology, 12,* 279–300.

Watson, D., Clark, L. A., & Tellegen, A. (1988). Development and validation of brief measures of positive and negative affect: The PANAS scales. *Journal of Personality and Social Psychology, 54,* 1063–1070.

Xanthopoulou, D., Bakker, A. B., Demerouti, E., & Schaufeli, W. B. (2009a). Reciprocal relationships between job resources, personal resources, and work engagement. *Journal of Vocational Behavior, 74,* 235–244.

Xanthopoulou, D., Bakker, A. B., Demerouti, E., & Schaufeli, W. B. (2009b). Work engagement and financial returns: A diary study on the role of job and personal resources. *Journal of Occupational and Organizational Psychology, 82,* 183–200.

Do you want me to be perfect? Two longitudinal studies on socially prescribed perfectionism, stress and burnout in the workplace

Julian H. Childs[a] and Joachim Stoeber[b]

[a]Centre for Health Services Studies, University of Kent, Canterbury, UK; [b]School of Psychology, University of Kent, Canterbury, UK

Stress and burnout in the workplace have a negative impact not only on individuals but also on organizations, clients and customers and are estimated to be of high cost to a country's economy. To help identify employees at high risk, it is important to know what individual differences contribute to stress and burnout. Two longitudinal studies were conducted to examine whether individual differences in socially prescribed perfectionism (individuals' perceptions that others have perfectionistic expectations of them) contribute to employees' role stress and predict increases in burnout symptoms (exhaustion, cynicism and inefficacy). Study 1 investigated 69 healthcare service provision employees in the UK over a six-month interval, and Study 2 investigated 195 school teachers in the UK over a three-month interval. In both studies, socially prescribed perfectionism predicted increases in role stress and inefficacy over time. Moreover, in Study 2, socially prescribed perfectionism also predicted increases in exhaustion and cynicism over time. The findings indicate that individual differences in socially prescribed perfectionism may be a contributing factor to stress and burnout in the workplace.

Introduction

Stress is a significant occupational hazard that can impair employees' physical health, psychological wellbeing and performance (e.g. Griffin & Clarke, 2011). Alongside depression and anxiety, stress is one of the leading causes of employee absenteeism. In the United Kingdom for example, stress is estimated to cause over 11 million lost working days, costing society £3.7 (US $5.8) billion per year (Health and Safety Executive, 1999, 2010). In the National Health Service (NHS) alone, the largest employer in Europe, stress is estimated to account for over 30% of sickness absence, costing taxpayers £300-400 (US $470-630) million per year (NHS Employers, 2010; NHS Jobs, 2009). Moreover, in the education sector, stress alongside depression and anxiety is the leading cause of employee absenteeism, and school teachers have been shown to experience particularly high levels of stress on the job (Health and Safety Executive, 2000).

Role stress is one of the most widely researched forms of job stress (e.g. Jackson & Schuler, 1985). Role stress has two main aspects: role conflict and role ambiguity

(Katz & Kahn, 1978; Rizzo, House, & Lirtzman, 1970). Role conflict occurs when employees are required to perform two or more incompatible behaviours, and role ambiguity occurs when employees are unclear as to what behaviours they are required to perform (Katz & Kahn, 1978). Role conflict and role ambiguity have been shown to be associated with higher levels of burnout and to predict increases in burnout over time (e.g. Lee & Ashforth, 1993; Örtqvist & Wincent, 2010; Peiró, González-Romá, Tordera, & Mañas, 2001; also see Cordes & Dougherty, 1993; Lee & Ashforth, 1996; Örtqvist & Wincent, 2006). Role conflict and role ambiguity also represent job demands in the job demands-resources model of job stress and employee burnout (Bakker, Demerouti, de Boer, & Schaufeli, 2003; Demerouti, Bakker, Nachreiner, & Schaufeli, 2001).

Burnout is a psychological syndrome characterized by exhaustion, cynicism and inefficacy (Schaufeli, Leiter, Maslach, & Jackson, 1996). Exhaustion refers to a depletion of one's emotional resources; cynicism to a negative, detached, and depersonalized attitude towards one's work; and inefficacy to feeling incompetent at work and unable to solve problems that arise in one's work (Schaufeli et al., 1996; Schaufeli, Salanova, González-Romá, & Bakker, 2002). Although initially applied only to human service workers, burnout is now one of the most widely researched consequences of chronic and severe stress in employees from a range of different professions as well as students (e.g. Cooper, Dewe, & O'Driscoll, 2001; Schaufeli, Martínez, Pinto, Salanova, & Bakker, 2002).

Burnout has a negative impact on employees, organizations, clients and customers. Burnout has been associated with higher levels of physical ill-health, negative perceptions of job characteristics, working excessively and compulsively, absenteeism, turnover, insomnia, depression, alcohol and drug abuse, negative affect, and marital and family problems, and with lower levels of work morale, quality of patient care, and positive affect (Hakanen, Schaufeli, & Ahola, 2008; Maudgalya, Wallace, Daraiseh, & Salem, 2006; Schaufeli, Bakker, van der Heijden, & Prins, 2009; Schaufeli et al., 1996; Thoresen, Kaplan, Barsky, Warren, & de Chermont, 2003). In terms of performance, the component exhaustion has been consistently associated with lower levels of objective ratings of in-role job performance, organizational citizenship behaviour, and customer satisfaction (see Taris, 2006, for a review). In the education sector, school teachers are among those professionals with the highest levels of burnout on the job, and many teachers retire early because they feel burnt out (e.g. Cano-García, Padilla-Muñoz, & Carrasco-Ortiz, 2005; Enzmann & Kleiber, 1989; Farber, 1991; Hakanen, Bakker, & Schaufeli, 2006; Tang, Au, Schwarzer, & Schmitz, 2001).

Perfectionism, stress, and burnout

Research has shown that, in addition to contextual factors such as job demands and job resources (Demerouti et al., 2001), personality characteristics play an important role in employee stress and burnout and may help predict who is at risk for developing stress and burnout in the workplace (e.g. Bakker, Van der Zee, Lewig, & Dollard, 2006; Cano-García et al., 2005).

One personality characteristic that has been closely associated with individual differences in stress and burnout is perfectionism. Perfectionism is characterized by striving for flawlessness, setting exceedingly high standards for performance, and overly critical evaluations of one's behaviour (Flett & Hewitt, 2002; Frost, Marten, Lahart, & Rosenblate, 1990). Perfectionism is a common personality characteristic that can affect all domains of life but is most prevalent in the domain of work with 53% of people in a sample of internet users reporting that they are perfectionistic at work (Stoeber & Stoeber, 2009; see also Slaney & Ashby, 1996). Perfectionism has been shown to explain variance in work-related outcomes above and beyond higher order personality traits (Clark, Lelchook, & Taylor, 2010). Moreover, perfectionism can be expected to be associated with role stress because role conflict involves perceived discrepancies between performance and expectations and because role ambiguity involves unclear performance standards, both of which are central to perfectionism (Hewitt & Flett, 1991; Kahn, Wolfe, Quinn, Snoek, & Rosenthal, 1964; Rizzo et al., 1970; Shafran, Cooper, & Fairburn, 2002).

One of the most widely researched models of perfectionism is that of Hewitt and Flett (1991), which differentiates between two main forms of perfectionism: socially prescribed perfectionism and self-oriented perfectionism. Socially prescribed perfectionism comprises externally motivated beliefs that excessively high standards are expected by others and that acceptance by others is conditional on fulfilling these standards, and it is characterized by individuals' perceptions that others impose perfectionistic standards onto them. In contrast, self-oriented perfectionism comprises internally motivated beliefs that striving for perfection and being perfect are important, and it is characterized by having a "perfectionistic motivation" for oneself (Enns & Cox, 2002; Hewitt & Flett, 1991, 2004; Stoeber, Feast, & Hayward, 2009).

The present research focuses on socially prescribed perfectionism because socially prescribed perfectionism has been associated with higher levels of professional distress, intolerance of ambiguity, job dissatisfaction, and emotional, bio-behavioural, and physiological manifestations of stress whereas self-oriented perfectionism only showed associations with professional distress and intolerance of ambiguity (Flett, Hewitt, & Hallett, 1995; Wittenberg & Norcross, 2001). Also, in athletes, socially prescribed perfectionism has been associated with higher levels of burnout whereas self-oriented perfectionism was associated with lower levels (Appleton, Hall, & Hill, 2009; Hill & Appleton, 2011; Hill, Hall, Appleton, & Kozub, 2008; Hill, Hall, Appleton, & Murray, 2010). Three studies have examined the two forms of perfectionism and burnout in samples of employees from a range of occupations, and in these studies socially prescribed perfectionism was consistently associated with higher levels of burnout (Childs & Stoeber, 2010; Mitchelson & Burns, 1998; van Yperen, Verbraak, & Spoor, 2011). Only in one study (Childs & Stoeber, 2010) was self-oriented perfectionism associated with lower levels of two components of burnout: cynicism and inefficacy. To summarize, whereas socially prescribed perfectionism has been consistently positively associated with stress and burnout in samples of employees and athletes, self-oriented perfectionism has shown a mix of positive, negative and non-significant associations with those outcomes.

In addition to stress and burnout, socially prescribed perfectionism has also been shown to be consistently associated with a variety of indicators of psychological maladjustment such as anticipation of future hassles and negative social interactions, depression, various forms of anxiety, suicide ideation and suicide attempts, harsh self-criticism, exercise dependence and disordered eating, and martial maladjustment (Frost & DiBartolo, 2002; Goldner, Cockell, & Srikameswaran, 2002; Hall, Hill,

Appleton, & Kozub, 2009; Haring, Hewitt, & Flett, 2003; Hewitt & Flett, 1991, 2002; Hewitt, Flett, & Weber, 1994; Nepon, Flett, Hewitt, & Molnar, 2011; O'Connor, 2007; Stoeber et al., 2009; Tissot & Crowther, 2008).

Socially prescribed perfectionism is closely associated with maladjustment because socially prescribed perfectionists do not strive to attain their personal perfectionistic standards, but the perfectionistic standards that they believe others – such as managers, coworkers, customers, and students and their parents – impose on them. Socially prescribed perfectionism should be associated particularly with role stress since a role includes expectations from others, and both socially prescribed perfectionism and role stress are underpinned by social expectations (Kahn et al., 1964; Hewitt & Flett, 1991; Rizzo et al., 1970). For socially prescribed perfectionists, standards are not only excessively high but also integral to self-identity and self-worth since these individuals believe that acceptance and approval are conditional upon attaining others' standards (Hill, Hall, & Appleton, 2011). Hence, socially prescribed perfectionists face a paradox as they do not believe they can live up to others' high standards even though doing so is the very cornerstone of their self-worth (Hall, 2006; Hewitt & Flett, 1993). Correspondingly, socially prescribed perfectionism has been shown to be associated with beliefs that failure is associated with negative interpersonal consequences (Conroy, Kaye, & Fifer, 2007).

When socially prescribed perfectionists first experience role stress, they may engage in increased achievement-striving to compensate for the threat to self-worth (e.g. Hall, 2006; Hall, Hill, & Appleton, 2012; Hewitt & Flett, 1991, 1993, 2002; Shafran et al., 2002; Shafran, Egan, & Wade, 2010). However, increased achievement striving may be maladaptive in the long term as it might deplete resources, suggesting that socially prescribed perfectionists may experience increased role stress when they encounter subsequent role stressors. Role stressors may also signal negative interpersonal consequences to socially prescribed perfectionists as they believe that others will reject them. Hence, these perfectionists should experience not only high levels of role stress in response to role stressors but also high levels of strain (e.g. burnout) because of reduced self-worth and debilitating self-criticism.

The present research

So far, however, no study has employed longitudinal designs investigating whether socially prescribed perfectionism is a contributing factor to the development and maintenance of stress and burnout in the workplace. To our knowledge, all studies so far have investigated perfectionism, stress, and burnout using cross-sectional designs that only provide information on the co-occurrence of socially prescribed perfectionism, stress and burnout, but no information on whether socially prescribed perfectionism predicts *increases* in stress and burnout. This is a general limitation of studies investigating personality and burnout because the majority only employ cross-sectional correlational designs (see, e.g. the meta-analysis by Alarcon, Eschleman, & Bowling, 2009) which do not provide any indication of possible causal pathways between personality, stress and burnout compared to studies using longitudinal correlational designs (see also Taris, 2000).

The aim of the present research was therefore to investigate whether socially prescribed perfectionism is associated with increases in role stress and burnout in the workplace over time. To this end, two studies were conducted. Study 1 investigated employees working in healthcare service provision and used a longitudinal design with two measurement points six months apart. Study 2 investigated teachers and used a longitudinal design with two measurement points three months apart. In both studies, we expected socially prescribed perfectionism to predict longitudinal increases in role stress and burnout.

Study 1

Method

Participants

A sample of 116 administrative and managerial employees was recruited from a National Health Service Primary Care Trust in the South of England. Of these, 59% returned data for both measurement points that did not show multivariate outliers (see section entitled *Preliminary analyses*). Hence, the final sample used in our longitudinal analyses comprised $N = 69$ employees (14 male, 55 female). Mean age of employees was 41.0 years ($SD = 11.4$; range $= 19–61$ years). Mean time employees had worked in full-time employment was 18.3 years ($SD = 12.2$; range $= 0.2–48.0$ years) and mean time employees had been in their current job was 2.6 years ($SD = 4.5$; range $= 0.1–28.0$ years). Employees' job types were administrative assistant (7%), administrator (13%), senior administrator (16%), team coordinator (16%), team leader (5%), middle management (19%), and senior management (24%). Employees' highest level of completed education was middle school (8%), high school (10%), further education (16%), and university degree (66%).

Procedure and design

Employees were recruited via the staff's electronic newsletter and intranet site. Both informed consent form and questionnaire were presented on the organization's secure online questionnaire management system (OQMS). The study employed a longitudinal correlational design with two measurement points: Time 1 (T1) and Time 2 (T2). Employees were asked to complete the T1 questionnaire in August 2009 and the T2 questionnaire six months later (T2). The study was approved by the relevant ethics committees and followed the British Psychological Society's (2009) code of ethics and conduct.

Measures

To measure socially prescribed perfectionism, we used the respective 15-item scale (e.g. "People expect nothing less than perfection from me") from the Multi-dimensional Perfectionism Scale (MPS; Hewitt & Flett, 1991, 2004). In addition, we included the 15-item scale capturing self-oriented perfectionism (e.g. "I demand nothing less than perfection for myself") to examine if self-oriented perfectionism had any effects on role stress and burnout over and beyond socially prescribed perfectionism. To capture perfectionism at work, employees were asked to respond to the items regarding their work. Although there are questions regarding the factorial validity of the MPS scales (Cox, Enns, & Clara, 2002), both scales have demonstrated reliability and validity in numerous studies (see Hewitt & Flett, 2004, for a comprehensive review). Because of constraints in the organization's OQMS, we could not implement the MPS's original 7-point answer scale. Instead, employees responded to the items on a scale from 1 (*strongly disagree*) to 5 (*strongly agree*).

To measure role stress, we used the 14-item Role Stress Scale (RSS; Rizzo et al., 1970). Following previous research (e.g. Dale & Fox, 2008; Thomas & Lankau, 2009) we measured total role stress combining role conflict (eight items; e.g. "I receive incompatible requests from two or more people") and role ambiguity items (six items; e.g. "Clear, planned goals and objectives exist for my job," reverse-coded). The RSS is a widely used measure of work stress and has demonstrated reliability and validity in numerous studies (e.g. Dale & Fox, 2008; Thomas & Lankau, 2009). Employees responded to the items on a scale from 1 (*strongly disagree*) to 5 (*strongly agree*).

To measure burnout, we used the 16-item Maslach Burnout Inventory-General Survey (MBI-GS; Schaufeli et al., 1996) capturing exhaustion (five items; e.g. "I feel emotionally drained from my work"), cynicism (five items; e.g. "I doubt the significance of my work"), and inefficacy (six items; e.g. "I can effectively solve the problems that arise in my work," reverse-coded). The MBI-GS is a widely used measure of burnout across occupational groups and has demonstrated reliability and validity in numerous studies (see Schaufeli et al., 1996, for a review). Employees responded to the items on a scale from 1 (*never*) to 5 (*always*).

Preliminary analyses

For all measures, mean scores were computed by averaging responses across items (see Table 1). All scores showed Cronbach's alphas above the .70 recommended for research purposes (Nunnally, 1978), except T2 inefficacy (alpha = .68). To examine possible differences between employees who completed both questionnaires (T1 and T2) and employees who only completed the T1 questionnaire, we computed a MANOVA with T2 completion (completer vs. non-completer) as between-participants factor and the six T1 variables (socially prescribed perfectionism, self-oriented perfectionism, role stress, exhaustion, cynicism, inefficacy) as dependent variables. The test was non-significant with $F(6, 109) = 1.54$, *ns* indicating that employees who completed both questionnaires were not significantly different from employees who completed only T1. Because the study focused on longitudinal effects, the employees who only completed T1 were excluded from all further analyses. Next, as recommended by Tabachnick and Fidell (2007), data were screened for multivariate outliers regarding the 10 variables included in the longitudinal analyses (T1 socially prescribed and self-oriented perfectionism; T1 and T2 role stress, exhaustion, cynicism, and inefficacy). One employee showed a Mahalanobis distance larger than $\chi^2(10) = 29.59$, $p < .001$ and was excluded from all further analyses. Finally, we examined the data for possible gender differences by computing a Box's M test (see Tabachnick & Fidell, 2007). The test was non-significant, Box's $M = 90.41$, $F(55, 1861) = 1.14$, *ns*. Therefore data were collapsed across gender.

Analytic strategy

To examine the relationships between perfectionism, stress and burnout we conducted two sets of analyses. First, we computed bivariate correlations between

Table 1. Correlations and descriptive statistics.

	1	2	3	4	5	6	7	8	9	10	Study 1			Study 2		
											M	SD	α	M	SD	α
Perfectionism																
1. T1 SPP	—	.26*	.41***	.47***	.51***	.52***	.29*	.31**	.14	.33**	2.82	0.70	.87	4.53	0.96	.87
2. T1 SOP	.48***	—	−.10	.06	−.01	.08	−.19	.07	−.28*	−.02	3.62	0.67	.88	5.04	1.07	.92
Role stress																
3. T1 role stress	.50***	.17*	—	.64***	.65***	.53***	.54***	.44***	.38***	.43***	2.90	0.62	.80	4.74	1.00	.83
4. T2 role stress	.46***	.20**	.70***	—	.58***	.67***	.48***	.58***	.33**	.56***	2.69	0.64	.85	4.53	1.09	.87
Burnout																
5. T1 exhaustion	.50***	.23***	.63***	.56***	—	.79***	.77***	.59***	.25*	.55***	2.89	1.16	.94	5.70	1.40	.91
6. T2 exhaustion	.43***	.22***	.42***	.58***	.65***	—	.55***	.70***	.32**	.56***	2.75	1.01	.91	5.50	1.44	.93
7. T1 cynicism	.40***	.00	.45***	.42***	.59***	.49***	—	.66***	.26*	.48***	2.40	1.11	.88	4.52	1.72	.86
8. T2 cynicism	.39***	.01	.44**	.55***	.50***	.64***	.75***	—	.22	.62***	2.41	1.08	.95	4.78	1.65	.87
9. T1 inefficacy	.51***	.10	.52**	.41***	.50***	.41***	.54***	.48***	—	.45***	1.82	0.58	.81	3.43	1.64	.81
10. T2 inefficacy	.45**	.08	.41***	.49***	.37***	.41***	.46***	.57***	.70***	—	2.00	0.51	.68	3.35	1.60	.85

Note: Correlations for Study 1 ($N = 69$) are presented above the diagonal and correlations for Study 2 ($N = 195$) below the diagonal. All scores are mean scores, and in Study 1 employees responded to all items on a 5-point scale (see Study 1, Method) whereas in Study 2 teachers responded on a 7-point scale (see Study 2, Method). SPP = socially prescribed perfectionism, SOP = self-oriented perfectionism, α = Cronbach's alpha.
*$p < .05$; **$p < .01$; ***$p < .001$.

all variables. Second, we computed hierarchical regression analyses to examine whether perfectionism was associated with increases in role stress and burnout symptoms over time. For each outcome variable at T2 (role stress, exhaustion, cynicism, inefficacy) one model was tested, comprised of three steps (see Taris, 2000). In Step 1, we entered the outcome variable at T1 to control for baseline effects. In Step 2, to test our hypotheses, we entered T1 socially prescribed perfectionism to examine whether it would predict residual changes in the outcome variable from T1 to T2. In Step 3, to explore if self-oriented perfectionism had any additional effects, we entered T1 self-oriented perfectionism.

Results: Study 1

Bivariate correlations

Table 1 shows the bivariate correlations. In line with previous cross-sectional findings, socially prescribed perfectionism showed positive correlations with role stress, exhaustion and cynicism at T1, and with role stress, exhaustion, cynicism and inefficacy at T2. Self-oriented perfectionism showed a positive correlation with socially prescribed perfectionism at T1 and a negative correlation with inefficacy at T1.

Regression analyses

Table 2 shows the results of the regression analyses. As expected, socially prescribed perfectionism was associated with increased role stress over time. Employees high in socially prescribed perfectionism not only showed higher levels of role stress at T1 compared to employees low in socially prescribed perfectionism, but their level of role stress further increased over the six-month period. Moreover, socially prescribed perfectionism was associated with increased burnout over time. However, this effect was significant only for one burnout symptom: inefficacy. Although employees high in socially prescribed perfectionism did not show higher levels of inefficacy at T1 compared to employees low in socially prescribed perfectionism, their level of inefficacy increased over the six-month period. Self-oriented perfectionism did not have any effects on the T2 outcome variables over and beyond socially prescribed perfectionism.

Brief discussion: Study 1

The findings of Study 1 are the first to suggest that socially prescribed perfectionism may be a personality characteristic that contributes to the development of role stress and burnout in employees over time. Socially prescribed perfectionism in employees was not only cross-sectionally associated with higher levels of role stress and burnout, it was also longitudinally associated with increased levels of role stress and burnout.

Study 1, however, had a number of limitations. First, the findings regarding burnout were restricted to one aspect (inefficacy). Second, the reliability (Cronbach's alpha) of T2 inefficacy was lower than desirable. Moreover, and more importantly, the measure we used to assess inefficacy has been criticized because it is comprised of reverse-coded items only and thus captures efficacy (indicating high levels of job

Table 2. Regressions of perfectionism predicting role stress and burnout: Study 1.

| | T2 role stress | | Burnout | | | | | |
| | | | T2 exhaustion | | T2 cynicism | | T2 inefficacy | |
Steps and variables	ΔR^2	β	ΔR^2	β	ΔR^2	β	ΔR^2	β
Step 1: Baseline	.413***		.619***		.441***		.200***	
T1 outcome variable		.64***		.79***		.66***		.45***
Step 2: SPP	.050*		.018		.017		.074*	
T1 SPP[a]		.25*		.16		.13		.28*
Step 3: SOP	.002		.002		.026		.001	
T1 SOP		.05		.05		.18		.03

Note: $N = 69$. [a]$f^2 = .09$ for T2 role stress and .10 for T2 inefficacy (Cohen, 1988). SPP = socially prescribed perfectionism, SOP = self-oriented perfectionism.
*$p < .05$. **$p < .01$. ***$p < .001$.

engagement, not low levels of burnout) rather than inefficacy (see Schaufeli & Salanova, 2007, for details). Third, the longitudinal sample was rather small, comprising only 69 employees. Consequently, the study may have been "under-powered" (Maxwell, 2004), that is, have had insufficient statistical power to detect further effects of socially prescribed perfectionism on burnout such as effects on the other two aspects, exhaustion and cynicism. Finally, the sample comprised only employees working in healthcare provision. Therefore, it is unclear if the findings would generalize to other employees.

To address these limitations, we conducted a second study with a larger sample of employees working in the educational setting (school teachers) using a revised inefficacy scale comprised of items capturing inefficacy proper (rather than reversed-coded efficacy) to examine whether the findings of Study 1 could be replicated and extended in a larger longitudinal sample of employees working in a different setting.

Study 2

Method

Participants

A sample of 349 school teachers was recruited via the Teacher Support Network, an independent charity that provides information, advice, and support to teachers in the UK. Of these, 56% returned data for both measurement points that did not show multivariate outliers (see *Preliminary analyses* section). Hence, the final longitudinal sample comprised $N = 195$ school teachers (38 male, 157 female). Mean age of teachers was 44.5 years ($SD = 10.2$; range $= 22$–63 years). Mean time teachers had been teaching was 15.5 years ($SD = 10.6$; range $= 0.3$–40.3 years) and mean time teachers had been in their current job was 6.5 years ($SD = 6.0$; range $= 0.1$–33.0 years). Teachers' job types were teaching assistant (1%), supply teacher (3%), teacher (61%), subject coordinator (3%), departmental head (15%), deputy head teacher (7%), head teacher (5%), and 5% were unclassified. All teachers had a university degree.

Procedure and design

Teachers were recruited via an advertisement on the Teacher Support Network's electronic newsletter and website. Both informed consent form and questionnaire were presented on our University's secure OQMS. The study employed a longitudinal correlational design with two measurement points: Time 1 (T1) and Time 2 (T2). Teachers were asked to complete the T1 questionnaire in November 2009 and the T2 questionnaire three months later (T2), which spanned a busy teaching period during the academic year when teachers have little time for recovery. The time between measurement points was reduced because there was a high rate of attrition in Study 1, and shorter intervals reduce sample attrition (Burisch, 2002); moreover, both six- and three-month intervals have been employed in past research on the development of burnout (e.g. Leiter, 1990; Leiter & Durup, 1996). As an incentive to participate, teachers who completed both questionnaires were entered into a raffle with prizes of one £100 voucher (approx. US $160), one £50 voucher (US $80), and two £25 vouchers (US $40). The study was approved by the relevant ethics committee and followed the British Psychological Society's (2009) code of ethics and conduct.

Measures

To measure perfectionism, role stress, and burnout, we used the same measures as in Study 1 except that we used Schaufeli and Salanova's (2007) inefficacy subscale that captures inefficacy (four items; e.g. "In my opinion, I'm inefficient in my job") without employing reverse-coded items (cf. Study 1, *Measures*). In addition, as the questionnaire was presented on our University's secure OQMS, teachers were able to responded to the perfectionism and role stress items on the original 7-point scale from 1 (*strongly disagree*) to 7 (*strongly agree*), and to the burnout items on a 7-point scale from 1 (*never*) to 7 (*always*).

Preliminary analyses

For all scales, mean scores were computed by averaging responses across items (see Table 1). All scores showed Cronbach's alphas above .70. To examine possible differences between teachers who completed both questionnaires (T1 and T2) and teachers who only completed the T1 questionnaire, we computed a MANOVA with T2 completion (completer vs. non-completer) as between-participants factor and the six T1 variables as dependent variables. The test was non-significant with $F(6, 342) = 0.94$, *ns* indicating that teachers who completed both questionnaires were not significantly different from teachers who completed only T1. Teachers who only completed T1 were excluded from all further analyses. Next, data were screened for multivariate outliers regarding the ten variables included in our longitudinal analyses. Two teachers showed a Mahalanobis distance larger than $\chi^2(10) = 29.59$, $p < .001$ and were excluded from all further analyses. Finally, to examine possible gender differences, we computed a Box's M test. The test was non-significant with Box's $M = 79.58$, $F(55, 15028) = 1.30$, *ns* so data were collapsed across gender.

Results and brief discussion: Study 2

Bivariate correlations

Table 1 shows the bivariate correlations. As in Study 1, socially prescribed perfectionism again showed positive correlations with role stress, exhaustion, and cynicism at T1 and T2, in addition to inefficacy at T2. Moreover, expanding on the findings from Study 1, this time socially prescribed perfectionism also showed a positive correlation with inefficacy at T1 (whereas it showed a non-significant correlation in Study 1). Self-oriented perfectionism showed positive correlations with socially prescribed perfectionism at T1 and with role stress and exhaustion at T1 and T2.

Regression analyses

Table 3 shows the results of the regression analyses. Expanding on the findings of Study 1, socially prescribed perfectionism this time predicted increases in role stress and all three burnout symptoms: exhaustion, cynicism and inefficacy. Teachers high in socially prescribed perfectionism not only showed higher levels of role stress and burnout at T1 compared to teachers low in socially prescribed perfectionism, but their levels of role stress and burnout further increased over the three-month period. Teachers high in socially prescribed perfectionism felt more stressed and burnt out at the beginning of the study and these feelings increased in the course of the study – a busy teaching period in the academic year – suggesting that socially prescribed perfectionism may be a contributing factor to stress and burnout in teachers. As in Study 1, self-oriented perfectionism did not have any effects over and beyond socially prescribed perfectionism.

Using a larger sample of different employees (school teachers), Study 2 replicated all findings of Study 1 in that socially prescribed perfectionism was associated with longitudinal increases in role stress and inefficacy. In addition, expanding on the

Table 3. Regressions of perfectionism predicting role stress and burnout: Study 2.

| | T2 role stress | | Burnout | | | | | |
| | | | T2 exhaustion | | T2 cynicism | | T2 inefficacy | |
Steps and variables	ΔR^2	β	ΔR^2	β	ΔR^2	β	ΔR^2	β
Step 1: Baseline T1 outcome variable	.482***	.70***	.425***	.65***	.568***	.75***	.490***	.70***
Step 2: SPP T1 SPP[a]	.016*	.15*	.013*	.13*	.010*	.11*	.012*	.13*
Step 3: SOP T1 SOP	.001	.03	.001	.03	.002	−.06	.002	−.05

Note: $N = 195$. [a]$f^2 = .03$ for T2 role stress, .02 for T2 exhaustion, .02 for T2 cynicism, and .02 for T2 inefficacy (Cohen, 1988). SPP = socially prescribed perfectionism, SOP = self-oriented perfectionism. *$p < .05$. **$p < .01$. ***$p < .001$.

findings of Study 1, socially prescribed perfectionism was also associated with longitudinal increases in the other two burnout symptoms: exhaustion and cynicism.

General discussion

The aim of the present research was to investigate whether socially prescribed perfectionism in the workplace was associated with increases in role stress and burnout over time. To this end, two studies were conducted to investigate whether socially prescribed perfectionism predicted increases in role stress and burnout symptoms (exhaustion, cynicism and inefficacy) over time using longitudinal correlational designs with two measurement points. In Study 1, healthcare service provision employees were investigated over a six-month period, and in Study 2, school teachers were investigated over a three-month period.

As expected, socially prescribed perfectionism was associated with higher levels of role stress and burnout. Moreover, and more importantly, socially prescribed perfectionism was associated with increases in role stress and burnout over time. Employees high in socially prescribed perfectionism not only experienced higher levels of role stress and burnout symptoms at the beginning of the longitudinal studies compared to employees low in socially prescribed perfectionism, but they also showed an increase in role stress and burnout over the course of the studies. In Study 1, socially prescribed perfectionism was associated with increases in role stress and inefficacy. In Study 2, socially prescribed perfectionism was associated with increases in role stress and all three burnout symptoms: exhaustion, cynicism and inefficacy.

This research is the first to investigate longitudinal effects of perfectionism on stress and burnout in the workplace. The findings extend the literature on perfectionism at work by providing the first longitudinal results using a measure of socially prescribed perfectionism. By demonstrating that (1) healthcare provision employees and school teachers with higher levels of socially prescribed perfectionism showed increased levels of role stress and inefficacy longitudinally and (2) teachers with higher levels of socially prescribed perfectionism also showed increased levels of exhaustion and cynicism longitudinally, the present findings expand on previous evidence from cross-sectional studies that socially prescribed perfectionism is associated with higher levels of stress and burnout in employees (Childs & Stoeber, 2010; Flett et al., 1995; Mitchelson & Burns, 1998; van Yperen et al., 2011). Thus, socially prescribed perfectionism – a form of perfectionism characterized by externally motivated beliefs that excessively high standards are expected by others and that acceptance by others is conditional on fulfilling these standards – may be more than a correlate of stress and burnout. The findings suggest that socially prescribed perfectionism may be a personality characteristic that might contribute to the development and maintenance of role stress and burnout in the workplace.

The present research has some limitations. First, the research focused on role stress. While role stress is a central form of stress in the workplace (Jackson & Schuler, 1985; Katz & Kahn, 1978), it is not the only form of stress that employees experience. Moreover, role stress is an inherently social form of stress. Consequently, socially prescribed perfectionism, a form of perfectionism in which the social context plays a key role (Hewitt & Flett, 1991), may be particularly influential in social forms of stress such as role stress. Thus, future longitudinal studies on perfectionism and stress should include other indicators of stress such as those listed in the Job Content Questionnaire (Karasek, 1985) to explore if the present findings generalize to other forms of stress and also if socially prescribed perfectionism predicts higher levels of job demands and lower levels of job decision latitude (cf. Karasek, 1979; Karasek & Theorell, 1990).

Second, the present research used longitudinal designs with two measurement points and thus could not investigate longitudinal mediation effects (e.g. if role stress mediates the effect of socially prescribed perfectionism on burnout) for which longitudinal designs with three measurement points are required (Cole & Maxwell, 2003). Consequently, future studies would profit from employing three-wave longitudinal designs to investigate if increased role stress from Time 1 to Time 2 mediates the longitudinal effects of socially prescribed perfectionism at Time 1 on increased burnout from Time 1 to Time 3. In addition, future studies may profit from employing diary methods to examine the cognitive-behavioural pathway through which socially prescribed perfectionism is associated with increases in role stress and burnout (see Hewitt & Flett, 2002). Moreover, they could examine if state expressions of socially prescribed perfectionism, such as perfectionistic cognitions, alter as a result of changes in role stressors and levels of burnout (Flett, Hewitt, Blankstein, & Gray, 1998; Hewitt & Flett, 2002; Stoeber & Janssen, 2011). This could arise because increased achievement striving when stressors are first encountered may lead to lower levels of resources and higher levels of stress over time as perfectionists attend more and more to the discrepancy between their worsening performance and others' expectations (e.g. Hall, 2006; Hall et al., 2012; Hewitt & Flett, 1991, 1993; Shafran et al., 2002).

Finally, future research may profit from differentiating between different sources of socially prescribed perfectionism in the workplace. A study on perfectionism, stress and burnout in school teachers (Stoeber & Rennert, 2008) demonstrated that the sources of socially prescribed perfectionism make a difference: perceived pressure from their students to be perfect was related to higher levels of stress and perceived pressure to be perfect from students' parents to higher levels of burnout. In contrast, perceived pressure to be perfect from colleagues was related to lower levels of stress and burnout. Future studies should therefore include measures to investigate which sources of socially prescribed perfectionism in the workplace – namely, other employees in the perfectionists' role set (Kahn et al., 1964) such as the perfectionist's line manager, colleagues and "customers" (including clients, patients and students) – make the largest contribution to employee stress and burnout over time.

Despite these limitations, we believe that the present findings make a significant contribution to the literature on the role that personality plays in employee stress and burnout because they suggest that socially prescribed perfectionism is a personality characteristic that plays an important role in the development and maintenance of role stress and burnout in the workplace. In this study, employees who held strong beliefs that others had exceedingly high standards for them and expected them to be perfect not only experienced higher levels of role stress and burnout, they also showed increased role stress and burnout over time. Consequently, socially prescribed perfectionism may be a characteristic that managers should pay more attention to as it might present a risk not just to employees' mental health and wellbeing but also to the organization's ability to have employees deliver their services to the high standards that others (e.g. management, staff, clients and customers) expect.

References

Alarcon, G., Eschleman, K. J., & Bowling, N. A. (2009). Relationships between personality variables and burnout: A meta-analysis. *Work & Stress, 23,* 244–263.

Appleton, P. R., Hall, H. K., & Hill, A. P. (2009). Relations between multidimensional perfectionism and burnout in junior-elite male athletes. *Psychology of Sport and Exercise, 10,* 457–465.

Bakker, A. B., Demerouti, E., de Boer, E., & Schaufeli, W. B. (2003). Job demands and job resources as predictors of absence duration and frequency. *Journal of Vocational Behavior, 62,* 341–356.

Bakker, A. B., Van der Zee, K. I., Lewig, K. A., & Dollard, M. F. (2006). The relationship between the Big Five personality factors and burnout: A study among volunteer counselors. *Journal of Social Psychology, 146,* 31–50.

British Psychological Society. (2009). *Code of ethics and conduct.* London: Author.

Burisch, M. (2002). A longitudinal study of burnout: The relative importance of dispositions and experiences. *Work & Stress, 16,* 1–17.

Cano-García, F. J., Padilla-Muñoz, E. M., & Carrasco-Ortiz, M. Á. (2005). Personality and contextual variables in teacher burnout. *Personality and Individual Differences, 38,* 929–940.

Childs, J. H., & Stoeber, J. (2010). Self-oriented, other-oriented, and socially prescribed perfectionism in employees: Relationships with burnout and engagement. *Journal of Workplace Behavioral Health, 25,* 269–281.

Clark, M. A., Lelchook, A. M., & Taylor, M. L. (2010). Beyond the big five: How narcissism, perfectionism, and dispositional affect relate to workaholism. *Personality and Individual Differences, 48,* 786–791.

Cohen, J. (1988). *Statistical power analysis for the behavioral sciences* (2nd ed.). Mahwah, NJ: Lawrence Erlbaum Associates.

Cole, D. A., & Maxwell, S. E. (2003). Testing meditational models with longitudinal data: Questions and tips in the use of structural equation modeling. *Journal of Abnormal Psychology, 112,* 558–577.

Conroy, D. E., Kay, M. P., & Fifer, A. M. (2007). Cognitive links between fear of failure and perfectionism. *Journal of Rational-Emotive & Cognitive-Behavior Therapy, 25,* 237–253.

Cooper, C. L., Dewe, P. J., & O'Driscoll, M. P. (2001). *Organizational stress: A review and critique of theory, research, and applications.* London: Sage.

Cordes, C. L., & Dougherty, T. W. (1993). A review and integration of research on job burnout. *Academy of Management Review, 18,* 621–656.

Cox, B. J., Enns, M. W., & Clara, I. P. (2002). The multidimensional structure of perfectionism in clinically distressed and college student samples. *Psychological Assessment, 14,* 365–373.

Dale, K., & Fox, M. L. (2008). Leadership style and organizational commitment: Mediating effect of role stress. *Journal of Managerial Issues, 20,* 109–130.

Demerouti, E., Bakker, A. B., Nachreiner, F., & Schaufeli, W. B. (2001). The job demands-resources model of burnout. *Journal of Applied Psychology, 86,* 499–512.

Enns, M. W., & Cox, B. J. (2002). The nature and assessment of perfectionism: A critical analysis. In G. L. Flett & P. L. Hewitt (Eds.), *Perfectionism* (pp. 33–62). Washington, DC: APA.

Enzmann, D., & Kleiber, D. (1989). *Helfer-Leiden: Streß und Burnout in psychosozialen Berufen* [When helpers suffer: Stress and burnout in psycho-social professions]. Heidelberg: Asanger.

Farber, B. A. (1991). *Crisis in education: Stress and burnout in the American teacher.* San Francisco, CA: Jossey-Bass.

Flett, G. L., & Hewitt, P. L. (2002). Perfectionism and maladjustment: An overview of theoretical, definitional, and treatment issues. In P. L. Hewitt & G. L. Flett (Eds.), *Perfectionism* (pp. 5–31). Washington, DC: APA.

Flett, G. L., Hewitt, P. L., Blankstein, K. R., & Gray, L. (1998). Psychological distress and the frequency of perfectionistic thinking. *Journal of Personality and Social Psychology, 75*, 1363–1381.

Flett, G. L., Hewitt, P. L., & Hallett, C. J. (1995). Perfectionism and job stress in teachers. *Canadian Journal of School Psychology, 11*, 32–42.

Frost, R. O., & DiBartolo, P. M. (2002). Perfectionism, anxiety, and obsessive-compulsive disorder. In G. L. Flett & P. L. Hewitt (Eds.), *Perfectionism* (pp. 341–372). Washington, DC: APA.

Frost, R. O., Marten, P., Lahart, C., & Rosenblate, R. (1990). The dimensions of perfectionism. *Cognitive Therapy and Research, 14*, 449–468.

Goldner, E. M., Cockell, S. J., & Srikameswaran, S. (2002). Perfectionism and eating disorders. In G. L. Flett & P. L. Hewitt (Eds.), *Perfectionism* (pp. 319–340). Washington, DC: APA.

Griffin M. A., & Clarke, S. (2011). Stress and well-being at work. In S. Zedeck (Ed.), *APA handbook of industrial and organizational psychology: Maintaining, expanding, and contracting the organization* (Vol. 3, pp. 359–397). Washington DC: APA.

Hakanen, J. J., Bakker, A. B., & Schaufeli, W. B. (2006). Burnout and work engagement among teachers. *Journal of School Psychology, 43*, 495–513.

Hakanen, J. J., Schaufeli, W. B., & Ahola, K. (2008). The Job Demands-Resources model: A three-year cross-lagged study of burnout, depression, commitment, and work engagement. *Work & Stress, 22*, 224–241.

Hall, H. K. (2006). Perfectionism: A hallmark quality of world class performers, or a psychological impediment to athletic development? In D. Hackfort & G. Tenenbaum (Eds.), *Perspectives on sport and exercise psychology* (Vol. 1, pp. 178–211). Oxford: Meyer & Meyer Sport.

Hall, H. K., Hill, A. P., & Appleton, P. R. (2012). Perfectionism: A foundation for sporting excellence or an uneasy pathway toward purgatory? In G. C. Roberts & D. Treasure (Eds.), *Advances in motivation in sport and exercise* (3rd ed., pp. 129–168). Leeds: Human Kinetics.

Hall, H. K., Hill, A. P., Appleton, P. R., & Kozub, S. A. (2009). The mediating influence of unconditional self-acceptance and labile self-esteem on the relationship between multidimensional perfectionism and exercise dependence. *Journal of Abnormal Psychology of Sport and Exercise, 10*, 35–44.

Haring, M., Hewitt, P. L., & Flett, G. L. (2003). Perfectionism, coping, and quality of intimate relationships. *Journal of Marriage and Family, 65*, 143–158.

Health and Safety Executive. (1999). *The costs to Britain of workplace and work-related ill health in 1995/96* (2nd ed.). Norwich: HSE Books.

Health and Safety Executive. (2000). *The scale of occupational stress: A further analysis of the impact of demographic factors and type of job.* Suffolk: HSE Books.

Health and Safety Executive. (2010). *Self-reported work-related illness and workplace injuries in 2008/2009: Results from the Labour Force Survey.* Suffolk: HSE Books.

Hewitt, P. L., & Flett, G. L. (1991). Perfectionism in the self and social contexts: Conceptualization, assessment, and association with psychopathology. *Journal of Personality and Social Psychology, 60*, 456–470.

Hewitt, P. L., & Flett, G. L. (1993). Dimensions of perfectionism, daily stress, and depression: A test of the specific vulnerability hypothesis. *Journal of Abnormal Psychology, 102*, 58–65.

Hewitt, P. L., & Flett, G. L. (2002). Perfectionism and stress processes in psychopathology. In G. L. Flett & P. L. Hewitt (Eds.), *Perfectionism* (pp. 255–284). Washington, DC: APA.

Hewitt, P. L., & Flett, G. L. (2004). *Multidimensional Perfectionism Scale (MPS): Technical manual.* Toronto: Multi-Health Systems.

Hewitt, P. L., Flett, G. L., & Weber, C. (1994). Dimensions of perfectionism and suicide ideation. *Cognitive Therapy and Research, 18*, 439–460.

Hill, A. P., & Appleton, P. R. (2011). The predictive ability of the frequency of perfectionistic cognitions, self-oriented perfectionism and socially prescribed perfectionism in relation to symptoms of burnout in youth rugby players. *Journal of Sports Sciences, 29*, 695–703.

Hill, A. P., Hall, H. K., & Appleton, P. R. (2011). The relationship between multidimensional perfectionism and contingencies of self-worth. *Personality and Individual Differences, 50*, 238–242.

Hill, A. P., Hall, H. K., Appleton, P. R., & Kozub, S. A. (2008). Perfectionism and burnout in junior elite soccer players: The mediating influence of unconditional self-acceptance. *Psychology of Sport and Exercise, 9*, 630–644.

Hill, A. P., Hall, H. K., Appleton, P. R., & Murray, J. J. (2010). Perfectionism and burnout in canoe polo and kayak slalom athletes: The mediating influence of validation and growth-seeking. *The Sport Psychologist, 24*, 16–34.

Jackson, S. E., & Schuler, R. S. (1985). A meta-analysis and conceptual critique of research on role ambiguity and role conflict in work settings. *Organizational Behavior and Human Decision Processes, 36*, 16–78.

Kahn, R. L., Wolfe, D. M., Quinn, R. P., Snoek, J. D., & Rosenthal, R. A. (1964). *Organizational stress: Studies in role conflict and ambiguity.* New York, NY: John Wiley & Sons.

Karasek, R. A. (1979). Job demands, job decision latitude, and mental strain: Implications for job redesign. *Administrative Science Quarterly, 24*, 285–308.

Karasek, R. A. (1985). *Job content questionnaire and user's guide* (revision 1.1). Lowell: University of Massachusetts Lowell, Job Content Questionnaire Centre.

Karasek, R. A., & Theorell, T. (1990). *Healthy work: Stress, productivity, and the reconstruction of working life.* New York, NY: Basic Books.

Katz, D., & Kahn, R. L. (1978). *The social psychology of organizations.* New York, NY: Wiley.

Lee, R. T., & Ashforth, B. E. (1993). A longitudinal study of burnout among supervisors and managers: Comparisons between the Leiter and Maslach (1988) and Golembiewski et al. (1986) models. *Organizational Behavior and Human Decision Processes, 54*, 369–398.

Lee, R. T., & Ashforth, B. E. (1996). A meta-analytic examination of the correlates of the three dimensions of job burnout. *Journal of Applied Psychology, 81*, 123–133.

Leiter, M. P. (1990). The impact of family resources, control coping, and skill utilization on the development of burnout: A longitudinal study. *Human Relations, 43*, 1067–1083.

Leiter, M. P., & Durup, M. J. (1996). Work, home, and in between: A longitudinal study of spillover. *Journal of Applied Behavioral Science, 32*, 29–47.

Maudgalya, T., Wallace, S., Daraiseh, N., & Salem, S. (2006). Workplace stress factors and 'burnout' among information technology professionals: A systematic review. *Theoretical Issues in Ergonomics Science, 7*, 285–297.

Maxwell, S. E. (2004). The persistence of underpowered studies in psychological research: Causes, consequences, and remedies. *Psychological Methods, 9*, 147–163.

Mitchelson, J. K., & Burns, L. R. (1998). Career mothers and perfectionism: Stress at work and at home. *Personality and Individual Differences, 25*, 477–485.

Nepon, T., Flett, G. L., Hewitt, P. L., & Molnar, D. S. (2011). Perfectionism, negative social feedback, and interpersonal rumination in depression and social anxiety. *Canadian Journal of Behavioural Science, 43*, 297–308.

NHS Employers. (2010). *Stress.* Retrieved from http://bit.ly/lUtfMq

NHS Jobs. (2009). *The NHS—a rewarding place to work.* Retrieved from http://bit.ly/buvz89

Nunnally, J. C. (1978). *Psychometric theory.* New York, NY: McGraw-Hill.

O'Connor, R. C. (2007). The relations between perfectionism and suicidality: A systematic review. *Suicide and Life-Threatening Behavior, 37*, 698–714.

Örtqvist, D., & Wincent, J. (2006). Prominent consequences of role stress: A meta-analytic review. *International Journal of Stress Management, 13*, 399–422.

Örtqvist, D., & Wincent, J. (2010). Role stress, exhaustion, and satisfaction: A cross-lagged structural equation modeling approach supporting Hobfoll's loss spirals. *Journal of Applied Social Psychology, 40*, 1357–1384.

Peiró, J. M., González-Romá, V., Tordera, N., & Mañas, M. A. (2001). Does role stress predict burnout over time among health care professionals? *Psychology and Health, 16*, 511–525.

Rizzo, J. R., House, R. J., & Lirtzman, S. I. (1970). Role conflict and ambiguity in complex organisations. *Administrative Science Quarterly, 15*, 150–163.

Schaufeli, W. B., Bakker, A. B., van der Heijden, F. M. M. A., & Prins, J. T. (2009). Workaholism among medical residents: It is the combination of working excessively and compulsively that counts. *International Journal of Stress Management, 16*, 249–272.

Schaufeli, W. B., Leiter, M. P., Maslach, C., & Jackson, S. E. (1996). The Maslach Burnout Inventory—General survey. In C. Maslach, S. E. Jackson, & M. P. Leiter (Eds.), *MBI manual* (3rd ed., pp. 22–26). Palo Alto, CA: Consulting Psychologists Press.

Schaufeli, W. B., Martínez, I. M., Pinto, A. M., Salanova, M., & Bakker, A. B. (2002). Burnout and engagement in university students: A cross-national study. *Journal of Cross-Cultural Psychology, 33*, 464–481.

Schaufeli, W. B., & Salanova, M. (2007). Efficacy or inefficacy, that's the question: Burnout and work engagement, and their relationships with efficacy beliefs. *Anxiety, Stress, & Coping, 20*, 177–196.

Schaufeli, W. B., Salanova, M., González-Romá, V., & Bakker, A. B. (2002). The measurement of engagement and burnout: A confirmative analytic approach. *Journal of Happiness Studies, 3*, 71–92.

Shafran, R., Cooper, Z., & Fairburn, C. G. (2002). Clinical perfectionism: A cognitive-behavioural analysis. *Behaviour Research and Therapy, 40*, 773–791.

Shafran, R., Egan, S., & Wade, T. (2010). *Overcoming perfectionism*. London: Constable & Robinson.

Slaney, R. B., & Ashby, J. S. (1996). Perfectionists: Study of a criterion group. *Journal of Counseling and Development, 74*, 393–398.

Stoeber, J., Feast, A. R., & Hayward, J. A. (2009). Self-oriented and socially prescribed perfectionism: Differential relationships with intrinsic and extrinsic motivation and test anxiety. *Personality and Individual Differences, 47*, 423–428.

Stoeber, J., & Janssen, D. P. (2011). Perfectionism and coping with daily failure: Positive reframing helps achieve satisfaction at the end of the day. *Anxiety, Stress, & Coping, 24*, 477–497.

Stoeber, J., & Rennert, D. (2008). Perfectionism in school teachers: Relations with stress appraisals, coping styles, and burnout. *Anxiety, Stress, & Coping, 21*, 37–53.

Stoeber, J., & Stoeber, F. S. (2009). Domains of perfectionism: Prevalence and relationships with perfectionism, gender, age, and satisfaction with life. *Personality and Individual Differences, 46*, 530–535.

Tabachnick, B. G., & Fidell, L. S. (2007). *Using multivariate statistics* (5th ed.). Boston, MA: Pearson.

Tang, C. S.-K., Au, W.-T., Schwarzer, R., & Schmitz, G. (2001). Mental health outcomes of job stress among Chinese teachers: Role of stress resource factors and burnout. *Journal of Organizational Behavior, 22*, 887–901.

Taris, T. W. (2000). *A primer in longitudinal analysis*. Thousand Oaks, CA: Sage.

Taris, T. W. (2006). Is there a relationship between burnout and objective performance? A critical review of 16 studies. *Work & Stress, 20*, 316–334.

Thomas, C. H., & Lankau, M. J. (2009). Preventing burnout: The effects of LMX and mentoring on socialization, role stress, and burnout. *Human Resource Management, 20*, 417–432.

Thoresen, C. J., Kaplan, S. A., Barsky, A. P., Warren, C. R., & de Chermont, K. (2003). The affective underpinnings of job perceptions and attitudes: A meta-analytic review and integration. *Psychological Bulletin, 129*, 914–945.

Tissot, A. M., & Crowther, J. H. (2008). Self-oriented and socially prescribed perfectionism: Risk factors within an integrative model for bulimic symptomatology. *Journal of Social and Clinical Psychology*, *27*, 734–755.

van Yperen, N. W., Verbraak, M., & Spoor, E. (2011). Perfectionism and clinical disorders among employees. *Personality and Individual Differences*, *50*, 1126–1130.

Wittenberg, K. J., & Norcross, J. C. (2001). Practitioner perfectionism: Relationship to Ambiguity tolerance and work satisfaction. *Journal of Clinical Psychology*, *57*, 1543–1550.

A participative intervention to improve employee well-being in knowledge work jobs: A mixed-methods evaluation study

Ole Henning Sørensen[a] and David Holman[b]

[a]Department of Business and Management, Aalborg University, Aalborg, Denmark; [b]Manchester Business School, The University of Manchester, Manchester, UK

Many workers are employed in knowledge work (i.e. cognitively demanding jobs involving knowledge, such as IT engineers, academics and accountants). Using a mixed-methods approach, this study evaluated a participative organizational-level occupational health intervention designed to improve working conditions and psychological well-being of knowledge workers across six organizations in Denmark. The intervention was conducted over 14 months, including the planning, implementation and evaluation phases. Quantitative surveys were conducted at two time points (Ns: Time 1 = 157, Time 2 = 154, Time 1/2 = 99), and interviews and workshops were conducted at various stages. The qualitative evaluation showed that participants implemented relational and work process initiatives in response to concerns about task uncertainty, task ambiguity, job complexity and task interdependencies. The quantitative evaluation showed significant improvements in relational job characteristics and burnout. The scale of implementation depended upon employee commitment, timely support from senior management, provision of information, change process expertise, and appreciation of the social meanings and relational implications of job change initiatives. The study illuminates the challenges of job redesign in knowledge work jobs and shows that certain strategies (e.g. enriching job discretion) may not be suitable in such jobs because they may increase already problematic levels of task uncertainty and ambiguity.

Introduction

Knowledge work jobs, in which the primary task is the acquisition, creation and application of knowledge, can be motivating and rewarding. However, they can also be experienced as stressful (Grönlund, 2007; McClenahan, Giles, & Mallett, 2007). Preventing stress in knowledge work jobs is important, as they constitute a significant proportion of jobs in many developed economies (Brinkley, Fauth, Mahdon, & Theodoropoulou, 2010; Davenport, 2005) and may constitute up to 25% of jobs in Denmark, where this study was conducted (Rugulies, Martin, Garde, Persson, & Albertsen, 2012). One means of alleviating stress in knowledge work jobs is an organizational-level occupational health (OL-OH) intervention that seeks to change the contextual antecedents of stress, e.g. job and social characteristics (Semmer, 2006). The very few published studies of OL-OH interventions in knowledge work jobs have produced inconsistent findings (Bond & Bunce, 2001; Landsbergis & Vivona-Vaughan, 1995). The failure to find consistent evidence of beneficial effects may be a result of the difficulties associated with finding better alternatives to organizing knowledge work jobs, or it may be a result of issues arising during the implementation of such changes, e.g. lack of process support from senior management (Nielsen, Taris, & Cox, 2010).

Detailed information on the challenges of implementing OL-OH interventions in knowledge work is lacking from current studies but can be obtained through the use of longitudinal, mixed-method designs. Such designs have the advantage of being able to evaluate the extent of change and explain why changes did or did not occur. The aims of this paper are to examine how OL-OH initiatives can benefit knowledge workers and to shed light on the implementation factors that shape the success of such initiatives in knowledge work jobs. To meet these aims, the paper reports on a longitudinal mixed-methods evaluation of a participative OL-OH intervention in knowledge work jobs. As such, the paper contributes to our understanding of the general efficacy of OL-OH interventions in the particular context of knowledge work jobs and responds to calls for the increased use of mixed-methods designs in intervention research (Kompier, Geurts, Grundemann, Vink, & Smulders, 1998).

Knowledge work jobs and organizational-level occupational health interventions

According to Davenport, Javenpaa, and Beers (1996, p. 54), knowledge work jobs can be defined as those in which the primary task is the acquisition, creation, packaging or application of knowledge; the tasks tackled in knowledge work jobs are often highly complex and ambiguous with no simple solution (Alvesson, 1993) and require access to knowledge and resources that are socially distributed (Davenport, 2005). The nature of tasks in knowledge work jobs has implications for the characteristics of such jobs. The complexity of the task means that knowledge work jobs typically have a high level of cognitive demands and intellectual challenge, as well as a high level of task discretion and variety (DeFillippi, Arthur, & Lindsay, 2005; Drucker, 1993). The interdependent nature of knowledge work tasks means interruptions are frequent and that interaction and emotional demands can be high (Grant & Parker, 2009). Consequently, knowledge work jobs often combine high job resources (i.e. factors such as discretion and variety that facilitate the achievement of goals, promote learning and fulfil basic human needs) with high job demands (i.e. factors such as workload and interaction demands that require physical or psychological effort) (Demerouti, Bakker, Nachreiner, & Schaufeli, 2001). High levels of job resources can improve well-being and reduce stress, as they enhance the ability of the person to manage job demands (Humphrey, Nahrgang, & Morgeson, 2007; Karasek & Theorell, 1990) and research evidence supports the view that jobs which combine high job resources with moderate to high job demands (i.e. active jobs) typically have higher levels of well-being than jobs with other combinations of resources and demands, e.g. high demands, low resources (de Lange, Taris, Kompier, Houtman, & Bongers, 2003).

Although knowledge work jobs might typically combine high job resources and high demands – and can therefore be expected to promote employee well-being – studies indicate that knowledge work jobs can be stressful (McClenahan et al., 2007). Possible reasons for this include high job demands that outstrip the ability of knowledge workers to cope (Grönlund, 2007), long working hours which make it difficult to reconcile home and work requirements (Kinman & Jones, 2008) and high task uncertainty that makes it difficult to assess goal progress (McGrath, 1976). Another reason may be that the very high levels of job resources in knowledge work jobs require much mental effort (Baumeister, Vohs, & Tice, 2007) and therefore act as a chronic stressor (Gardner & Cummings, 1988). For example, Xie and Johns (1995) found a curvilinear relationship between job scope (a combined measure of five job resources: high control, skill variety, task identity, task significance and task feedback) and burnout, such that jobs with either a very low and or very high job scope were associated with higher burnout, whereas jobs with moderate levels of job scope were associated with lower levels of burnout.

An OL-OH intervention is one possible means of dealing with the problematic aspects of knowledge work jobs, and can be defined as planned, behavioural, theory-based change initiatives at the organizational level that aim to modify the contextual antecedents of job stress to improve the health and well-being of participants (Bambra, Egan, Thomas, Petticrew, & Whitehead, 2007; Egan et al., 2007). Systematic reviews of OL-OH interventions indicate their benefit to employee health, but the majority of these studies have been on low skill jobs and tend to focus on improving job resources by increasing task discretion (Bambra et al., 2007; Egan et al., 2007; Holman, Axtell, Sprigg, Totterdell, & Wall, 2010). However, as knowledge work jobs have high job resources, enhancing them in knowledge work jobs may be problematic as it may simply exacerbate job scope, task ambiguity and uncertainty (Xie & Johns, 1995).

We have identified only one longitudinal, mixed-methods OL-OH study on knowledge work jobs (Landsbergis & Vivona-Vaughan, 1995). In this study, the majority of employees in the sample were managers or professionals. As part of the intervention, employees developed seven organizational changes: regular meetings, improved filing procedures, a "quiet hour" without phone calls, drafting a department "policy and procedures" manual, a new phone answering system, more equal distribution of work, and more task variety. The changes that the knowledge workers sought to implement largely concerned the introduction of coordination rules, formal work procedures and feedback practices to improve planning. Yet no consistent differences between the intervention and control group was found. It was suggested that this was due to the short intervention period and concurrent externally introduced organizational changes. However, a lack of detailed description and analysis of the content, context and implementation of the change initiatives means that it is difficult to determine whether the changes were unsuccessful because they were poorly implemented or because they were inappropriate for knowledge workers, or both. Indeed, there is a growing recognition of the need to understand how the design and implementation of OL-OH interventions shapes their success or otherwise (Nielsen, Randall, Holten, & Rial González, 2010; Nielsen & Abildgaard, 2013) and various guidelines on the design of OL-OH intervention processes have been suggested. Kompier et al. (1998) proposed that OL-OH interventions should follow a stepwise and participative approach using a phase model for the intervention; while Nielsen et al.'s (2010) review of five European OL-OH models suggests five key phases. These are *preparation*: setting up the project and securing support; *screening*: determining the appropriate problems and solutions; *action planning*: designing the implementation and securing the necessary support; *implementation*: involving the right people and executing plans; and *evaluation*: learning from the course of events. From this it is evident that studies of OL-OH interventions in knowledge work jobs have not evaluated the quality of the intervention process. As such, the current occupational health literature does not address which sort of change initiatives are appropriate for knowledge work jobs and what issues might affect their implementation in OL-OH interventions. Furthermore, it has been argued that longitudinal mixed-methods designs are the most appropriate for assessing both the content and process of OL-OH interventions (Egan, Bambra, Petticrew, & Whitehead, 2009). The aims of the paper are therefore to use a longitudinal mixed-methods research design to examine how OL-OH initiatives can benefit knowledge workers and to shed light on the implementation factors that shape the success of OL-OH initiatives in knowledge work jobs.

Method

Participants and procedure

The aim of the OL-OH intervention in this study was to improve working conditions and employee well-being. It was conducted by staff from three Danish research institutions: The Technical University of Denmark (DTU), The National Research Centre for the Working Environment (NFA) and Copenhagen Business School (CBS). Using a purpose-designed sampling strategy, we obtained six organizational cases that varied according to ownership (public, private). The first two organizations participating in this study were departments in two large, private engineering companies working with environmental and plumbing consultancies, which we call EngWater (final $N = 19$ of 36) and EngPlumb, (final $N = 19$ of 30). The third case was a negotiation department within a national trade union for knowledge workers, which we call K-Union (final $N = 16$ of 33). The fourth and fifth cases were separate departments within a large municipal administration; one concerned with the municipality's finances (SocEco, final $N = 9$ of 15), the other being the political secretariat (SocSecr, final $N = 9$ of 13). They were treated as separate cases, as each had separate work tasks and they were not co-located. The sixth case was a design department of a toy manufacturer (TDesign, final $N = 26$ of 36). The response rates at both measurement occasions varied from 65% to 88%, and overall 61% of the participants who participated in the first baseline wave also participated in the follow-up wave (a table with more details can be requested from the authors). It was not possible to establish a control group, because all cases wanted to participate, or to use a waiting-list design due to funding constraints.

Study design

A complementary mixed-methods approach using qualitative and quantitative methodologies was adopted to evaluate the intervention (Nastasi et al., 2007). The entire intervention process lasted for 14 months. The first three months were the preparation phase, during which workshops and interviews were conducted. This was followed by an implementation phase of nine months, which started with a dialogue workshop focused on action planning by employees and included two progress meetings. Following the intervention there was a two-month evaluation phase, concluded by an evaluation workshop with all employees. A quantitative survey was conducted at two points during that time. Survey 1 was conducted two weeks before the end of the preparation phase. Survey 2 took place two weeks into the evaluation phase.

The intervention had four substantive phases: preparation, action planning, implementation and evaluation. The *preparation phase* of three months involved researchers informing employees about the intervention and gaining acceptance for it. This involved presentations to senior management, employee representatives and employees. Meetings with management and employee representatives dealt with budget and planning issues to secure the right conditions for the intervention and to establish rapport (Cox, Karanika, Griffiths, & Houdmont, 2007). At meetings with employees, the researchers presented the intervention and stressed the importance of the participatory approach.

The *action planning phase*, which included diagnosis of problems and the development of workplace initiatives, consisted of a four-hour workshop and subsequent time spent refining these initiatives. The workshop was facilitated by the researchers and was based on other participative change and job redesign methods (Holman et al., 2010). To ensure the best organizational and individual fit of the intervention (Randall & Nielsen, 2012), the workshop involved almost all employees and their manager discussing which work-related issues they found most salient with regard to well-being. Discussions were prompted by statements about work drawn from interviews conducted by the researchers with employees and managers in the preparation phase. Participating employees then prioritized the importance of these issues and developed the workplace change initiatives. Employee "initiative leaders" were appointed to refine the initiatives and to coordinate and drive the subsequent implementation process.

In the *implementation phase*, which lasted nine months, employees and initiative leaders were tasked with implementing changes, as well as discussing and assessing the progress of initiatives within normal meeting activities. Researcher-led workshops were conducted with the manager and initiative leaders at three and six months to discuss progress. The *evaluation phase* had one substantial activity, an evaluation workshop, where the employees presented their view of the changes and the researcher presented the results of the quantitative and qualitative evaluation for respondent validation.

Qualitative methodology

An aim of the qualitative methodology was to provide a detailed understanding of the intervention process and the workplace initiatives that arose from it. In particular, we sought a rich understanding of the intention, content, implementation and success (or otherwise) of each workplace initiative from the perspectives of various organizational stakeholders, e.g. employees, managers and local union representatives (Nielsen, Randall, & Albertsen, 2007; Randall, Nielsen, & Tvedt, 2009). A further aim was to obtain an understanding of the contextual factors (e.g. social relationships, administrative procedures, workplace changes) that might shape the intervention and its outcomes (Cordery, 1999; Landsbergis & Vivona-Vaughan, 1995). The results of the qualitative methodology were also used to inform the quantitative analysis and to explain the quantitative results.

For the qualitative evaluation, data were collected using different qualitative methods. Fifty-one semi-structured interviews with employees, initiative leaders and managers were conducted before, during and after the intervention. Participant observation was used in each of 30 workshops conducted in the various phases. Typically with one researcher facilitating the workshop and another observing and documenting electronically. Nine focus group interviews were also conducted during and after the intervention, with each group containing employees, initiative leaders and managers, with six to eight participants in each group. A research assistant took notes. The individual and focus group interviews concentrated on job characteristics, well-being, perception of the change initiative, implementation issues, and support from staff, management and employee representatives (Nielsen et al., 2007; Randall et al., 2009). Workshops and interviews were recorded when possible, all interviews were summarized, and interviews central for the analysis were transcribed. An electronic logbook was used to document occasions where the researchers intervened in the implementation process to assist the organization members, e.g. giving feedback on an initiative. Data were also collected from organizational documents and PowerPoint presentations.

Data from interviews, observation notes and logbook notes were entered into NVivo 8, which is a software package for qualitative data analysis, and analyzed using template analysis (Crabtree & Miller, 1999), with data from logbooks and observation notes analyzed first, followed by the interview data. The initial template categories were derived from relevant theoretical and empirical concepts (Gibbs, 2009) and included the phase of the project (preparation, action planning, implementation and evaluation), intervention properties (heading, aim, scale, status) and organizational and demographic attributes. The coding process involved reading and rereading the data, concept-driven coding of the text against initial template categories, open coding to develop new categories (the final template included additional sub-categories such as intervention type) and case comparison to understand distinctive case features (Gibbs, 2009). The data were also examined to provide examples of initiatives that were selected to illustrate the findings in this paper. Finally, for respondent validation and to assess the reliability of our analytical interpretations (Guest, MacQueen, & Namey, 2012), we presented the results of the analysis at workshops within each organization two to four months after the intervention. No objections were raised to the interpretations offered, which increased our confidence in the results of the qualitative data analysis.

Quantitative methodology

The aims of the quantitative methodology were twofold: to provide additional evidence on employee perceptions of the occupational health intervention process (e.g. knowledge of the intervention, degree of participation) and to provide evidence on whether the changes had influenced employee perceptions of job characteristics and well-being. A longitudinal survey conducted at two time points was used. The outcome variables were: job autonomy, workload, work tempo, relation quality, leader skill, leader support, co-worker support and burnout.

The Time 1 questionnaire was administered two weeks before the first workshop initiating the action planning phase. The Time 2 questionnaire was administered nine months later, in the evaluation phase. Previous studies have shown that changes in job characteristics can be detected three months after the end of an intervention and hence the choice of timescale is appropriate (Holman et al., 2010). The survey was administered by an employee within each respective organization. Employees completed the questionnaire in their own time and then sent it directly to the research team.

At Time 1, the survey was completed by 157 of 194 potential respondents across all six organizations, a response rate of 81%. There were 92 women and 65 men, the average age was 43.8 years and the average tenure was 10.1 years. At Time 2, all employees were given the opportunity to complete the survey, including those who did not respond at

Time 1 or had joined since Time 1. The survey was completed by 154 of 210 potential respondents across all six cases, a response rate of 73%. At Time 2 there were 94 women and 60 men, the average age was 41.5 years and the average tenure was 8.8 years. Ninety-nine employees, 63 women and 36 men, responded at Time 1 and 2.

Measures of process and outcome

Outcome measures were selected from the Copenhagen Psychosocial Questionnaire (Kristensen, Hannerz, Hogh, & Borg, 2005) to cover the three areas that we expected to change as a result of the intervention, i.e. job characteristics, relationship quality and employee well-being. These measures were used at both time points.

The three measures of *job characteristics* were: Job autonomy, a four-item measure concerning employees' control over their job task (T1 $\alpha = .65$; T2 $\alpha = .73$); Workload, a four-item measure assessing the amount of work (T1 $\alpha = .71$; T2 $\alpha = .71$); and Work tempo, a three-item measure of work pace (T1 $\alpha = .82$; T2 $\alpha = .80$).

The four measures of *relationship quality* were: Manager relationship quality, a three-item measure on the extent to which employees' work was recognized by managers (T1 $\alpha = .77$; T2 $\alpha = .67$); Leadership skills, a four-item measure of the extent to which the employee's leader was perceived to exhibit leadership skills, such as an ability to plan (T1 $\alpha = .71$; T2 $\alpha = .74$); Leader support, a three-item measure of social support provided by the employee's leader (T1 $\alpha = .70$; T2 $\alpha = .77$); and, a three-item measure of co-worker social support (T1 $\alpha = .72$; T2 $\alpha = .60$).

Job-related well-being was assessed using a four-item burnout measure concerning the extent to which an employee felt tired and exhausted from work in the last four weeks (T1 $\alpha = .84$; T2 $\alpha = .88$). All items were measured on 1–5 response scales ("*Always*" to "*Never/hardly ever*", "*To a very large extent*" to "*To a very small extent*" or "*All the time*" to "*Not at all*"). To aid interpretation, measures in the Copenhagen Psychosocial Questionnaire are transformed to scales of 1–100, as scale validation research shows that changes of three or above on this scale represent a clinically and phenomenologically meaningful level of change (Pejtersen, Bjørner, & Hasle, 2010). Scale means are reported in Table 1.

The survey also included measures of the intervention process. The intervention process measures were eight single items (see Table 2) on: knowledge and expectation of the intervention (e.g. What was your knowledge of the intervention?); participation (e.g. Were you involved in the intervention-related activities?) and support for the intervention from various stakeholders (e.g. Did senior management support the intervention?). All items were measured on 1–5 response scales ("*A very small extent*" to "*A very large extent*"). These items only appeared in the Time 2 survey.

Analyses

The data were analyzed in two ways. To examine differences between organizational cases with regard to perceptions of the intervention process, we used analysis of covariance (ANCOVA) to make comparisons between three groups of cases. On the basis of the qualitative evaluation, it was found that some organizational cases implemented many of the proposed changes, some implemented a few changes and some did not implement any of the proposed changes. On the basis of this, two cases were placed into a

Table 1. Correlations of job characteristics and well-being measures.

	T1		T2		Item scale	1	2	3	4	5	6	7	8	9	10	11	12
	Mean	SD	Mean	SD													
1. Job autonomy	50.9	15.7	51.6	15.3	0–100	.65\.73	−.09	.10	.47	.34	.37	.30	−.01	.04	−.09	.24	.23
2. Workload	55.3	16.1	53.9	14.8	0–100	−.22	.71\.71	.30	−.01	−.03	.23	.16	.20	.04	.06	−.07	−.05
3. Work tempo	70.0	15.1	67.3	15.1	0–100	−.15	.44	.82\.80	.08	.05	.20	.04	.16	−.06	.23	.08	−.11
4. Manager relationship quality	65.1	15.0	64.1	14.7	0–100	.16	−.33	−.12	.77\.67	.58	.57	.47	−.27	−.04	.11	.16	.17
5. Leader skill	58.6	14.0	57.8	13.5	0–100	.07	−.38	−.09	.39	.71\.74	.48	.42	−.14	−.04	.12	.05	.21
6. Leader support	62.4	17.2	59.4	18.3	0–100	.09	−.14	.16	.43	.53	.70\.77	.34	−.12	.06	.05	−.01	.08
7. Co-worker support	60.6	15.5	59.7	14.8	0–100	.04	.01	.02	.24	.12	.15	.72\.60	.08	−.19	.21	.23	.12
8. Burnout	34.6	17.6	34.1	18.9	0–100	−.17	.21	.05	−.18	−.10	−.07	−.14	.84\.88	−.28	.02	.12	−.18
9. Age	41.1	10.4	42.3	10.5	25–66	.19	.11	.04	−.05	.00	.10	−.20	−.23	–	.00	−.29	.06
10. Gender (male = 0)	0.64	0.48	0.64	0.48	0–1	−.11	.13	.22	.00	−.08	−.01	.09	−.07	.00	–	−.03	.02
11. Education (higher = 1)	0.85	0.36	0.85	0.36	0–1	.08	.05	.08	−.01	−.04	−.12	.20	.06	−.29	−.03	–	.11
12. Manager (yes = 1)	0.06	0.24	0.06	0.24	0–1	.21	.00	−.06	.14	−.08	−.10	.01	−.18	.06	.02	.11	–

Note: Time 1 correlations are shown below the diagonal and Time 2 above (N = 99). Correlations over .19 are significant at p < .05 and over .25 at p < .01. Cronbach's alpha T1\T2 are shown on the diagonal.

Table 2. Process evaluation: Means and implementation group differences (ANCOVA).

| | | Implementation group | | | | |
	All $N = 116$	High $N = 47$	Medium $N = 31$	Non $N = 38$	F	p
Knowledge and expectation						
1. Did you know about the project?	4.98	4.98	4.97	5.00	.35	*n.s*
2. Did you expect the project to be successful?	3.03	2.96	2.90	3.22	.49	*n.s*
Participation						
3. Have you been involved in project-related activities?	3.36	3.72	2.97	3.24	2.41	2
Provision of support for the intervention						
4. Did you support the project?	3.89	3.93	3.34	3.35	3.14	2
5. Did your colleagues support the project?	3.59	3.77	3.07	3.30	7.18	2
6. Did senior management support the project?	3.43	4.16	2.96	3.43	12.84	1
7. Did your department manager support the project?	3.93	3.29	3.72	3.65	3.68	2
8. Did you receive information on the intervention?	3.62	4.17	3.60	3.78	5.75	2

Note: *n.s.* = non-significant differences between groups; 1 = All groups were significantly different at $p < .01$; 2 = High-implementation group significantly different from other groups at $p < .05$, no significant difference between medium- and non-implementation groups. Measured at Time 2. Includes persons invited at both time points only (i.e. present during the entire intervention).

high-implementation group, two cases in a medium-implementation group and two cases in a non-implementation group. Further justification for this classification is given in the *Results* section, but the allocation criteria were assessments of the scale of the initiatives and the employees' support and involvement in the implementation. In the ANCOVA, the independent variable was implementation group membership, and the dependent variables were the eight intervention process measures, e.g. knowledge of the intervention. Control variables included gender, age and dummy variables for educational level (post-graduate education) and role (manager).

To analyze whether the intervention produced significant differences in change over time between the three groups (i.e. high-, medium- and non-implementation groups) with regard to job characteristics and well-being we used multilevel regression modelling, with measurement occasions (Level 1) nested within individuals (Level 2) (Raudenbush, Bryk, Cheong, & Congdon, 1999). The advantages of multilevel modelling over other techniques (e.g. RM-ANOVA) are that variance is correctly partitioned to the different levels and its robustness against violations of homoschedasticity and sphericity. This reduces Type 1 error rates and effect sizes can be estimated more accurately (Quené & van den Bergh, 2004).

We thought it would be useful to compare change between the three implementation groups, as it is reasonable to expect that greater changes will occur in the high- and medium-implementation groups, which had implemented changes, than in the non-implementation group that had not implemented any changes (Shadish & Cook, 1999). To compare differences in change over time between groups, we conducted a series of Level

1 moderation analyses. We first created dummy variables, one representing measurement time (i.e. pre- and post-intervention), three representing group membership, and three interaction terms representing the product of measurement time and group membership. We then conducted a series of regressions with measurement time, two group membership variables (e.g. high, medium) and the appropriate interaction terms (e.g. time x high implementation, time x medium implementation). The group membership variable not entered becomes the referent category. Repeating the analysis with each group as the referent enables change in the dependent variable to be compared across all groups. Random effects were fixed and individual controls (gender, age, educational level, role) were included as Level 2 predictors.

Results

We report the results of our analysis in two sections. The first section draws on both the qualitative and the quantitative analyses to provide an overview of the change initiatives developed in the intervention and to provide an evaluation of how the process and context of the intervention shaped the extent to which change initiatives were implemented. A key outcome of this is to show which change initiatives the knowledge workers found appropriate and the issues related to implementing them. Another outcome is that it supports the classification of the cases into three groups (high-, medium- and non-implementation group) that differed in terms of the type and extent of initiatives implemented and the speed of implementation. The second section draws on qualitative and quantitative analyses to provide an evaluation of how the employees' well-being and their perceptions of their job characteristics were affected by the intervention.

Evaluation of the intervention process

In this section we draw on interview, observational and survey data to evaluate how various factors (e.g. management support, employee participation) shaped the different phases of the intervention, i.e. preparation, action planning, implementation and evaluation. The evaluation phase was primarily a validation element in the project, and will not be described in detail.

Preparation phase. The aims of the preparation phase were to inform employees of the intervention and to gain their acceptance of its worth. The qualitative survey results (collected at Time 2, see Table 2) indicated that employees knew about the project to a large extent and expected the project to be successful to a moderate extent. In interviews, managers and employees stated that support at this stage was widespread. There were no significant differences between the cases with regard to employee's knowledge and expectations of the project or initial support, which suggests that any subsequent differences in implementation are unlikely to result from initial differences in these factors.

Action planning phase. The development of the workplace change initiatives started at dialogue workshops with discussions on the types of initiative that could be used to deal with problematic aspects of the job. Particular concern was expressed about high levels of task ambiguity and uncertainty, the technical and social complexity of certain projects, and working on multiple projects. These attributes were seen to cause difficulties with regard to crafting project boundaries, developing solutions at the right quality and price, prioritizing daily tasks, prioritizing projects and customers, and managing social contact (e.g. dealing with non-essential interruptions, carving out thinking time). These task attributes were also seen to affect working time (i.e. having to work long hours) and the ability to deliver projects on time.

Certain initiatives (e.g. management feedback, knowledge exchange), were proposed as ways of reducing ambiguity and uncertainty, and as a means of gaining a more concrete understanding of project boundaries, project solutions, task progress and task priorities. A department manager at EngWater explained that employees wanted feedback on "… how it really worked out, both regarding quality, time-use, and the time-horizon? Such questions were some of the most important elements". Other initiative ideas, concerned with managing working time and prioritizing tasks, were proposed in response to concerns about coping with task complexity, while managing social contacts and working time were seen as an important way of improving problem solutions and work efficiency. For example, initiatives aimed at the reduction of interruptions were developed in response to concerns about the difficulties of concentrating on demanding tasks during busy periods.

At the end of the workshop, the groups selected 30 change proposals that were thought to be most important (see Table 3, columns 3 and 4) and developed actions plans for each proposed change initiative. The initiatives were of two main types. *Relational initiatives* were primarily aimed at changing the nature of employee relationships through changes to feedback and the provision of social support. The different types (and number) of relational initiatives were: improving management feedback (3), improving feedback from colleagues (1), fostering a sense of community and improving communication between sub-units (2) and fostering engagement (1). *Work process initiatives* were primarily aimed at reducing task interruptions and workload to achieve better work processes and were: reducing interruptions (11), improving workload planning (7), improving meetings (3) and fostering creative processes (1). As each workplace underwent the same intervention process and developed several initiatives, it is unlikely that subsequent differences in implementation are a result of differences during this phase.

Implementation phase. Although actions plans had been developed for each change initiative, further work was needed to make initiatives workable. Some initiatives were harder to implement and some workplaces had greater difficulty implementing initiatives. Of the 30 proposed change initiatives, 16 were subsequently implemented (see Table 3, last column). Our process evaluation indicated that the cases differed according to the type, extent and speed of initiative implementation, such that there was a high-implementation group (EngWater and K-Union), a medium-implementation group (EngPlumb and SocEco) and a group that did not implement changes: a non-implementation group (T-Design and SocSecr).

With regard to differences between cases in the type of initiatives implemented, only EngWater and K-Union implemented *relational initiatives*. Employees at EngWater deve-oped and implemented a management feedback initiative that used a spreadsheet-based

Table 3.   Workplace initiatives proposed during workshops, and status of subsequent implementation.

Workplace	Type[a]	Initiative heading	Major objective	Scale[b]	Status[c]
High-implementation group					
EngWater	R	Management feedback	Better feedback	Large	Impl
	P	Registration of time	Fewer demands	Large	Impl
	P	Appropriate workload	Appropriate demands	Large	Impl
	P	Interruptions	Fewer interruptions	Large	Impl
K-Union	P	Better meetings	Less time wasted	Large	Impl
	R	Colleague feedback	Better feedback	Middle	Impl
	R	Management feedback	Better feedback/trust	N/A	No
	P	Time without interruptions	Fewer interruptions	N/A	No
	P	Fewer projects	Lower demands	N/A	No
Medium-implementation group					
EngPlumb	P	Planning meetings	Better plans	Middle	Impl
	P	Planning checklist	Better plans	Small	Impl
	P	Open office rules	Fewer interruptions	Small	Impl
	P	Telephone habits	Fewer interruptions	Middle	Impl
	P	Coloured signs	Fewer interruptions	Small	Impl
	P	Email norms	Fewer interruptions	N/A	No
	R	Management feedback	Better feedback	N/A	No
SocEco	P	Appropriate meetings	Better meetings	Middle	Impl
	P	Calendars and phones	Fewer interruptions	Small	Impl
	P	Monitoring of deadlines	Better workflow	Small	Impl
	P	Do-no-disturb signs	Fewer interruptions	N/A	No
	P	Less turnover	Less pressure	N/A	No
Non-implementation group					
SocSecr[d]	P	Turn-taking on meeting	Better meetings	Small	No
	R	Thematic seminars	Sense of community	Large	No
	R	Subunits communication	Better communication	Middle	No
	P	Email norms	Fewer interruptions	N/A	No
	P	Interruptions	Fewer interruptions	N/A	No
T-Design	P	Estimation of time	Better workflow	Large	No
	P	Interruptions	Fewer interruptions	N/A	No
	P	Creative processes	More creativity	N/A	No
	R	Engagement	Increase motivation	N/A	No

Note: [a]Change initiative was either relational (R) or work process related (P); [b]*Scale* refers to how many employees were affected by the initiative and how much; [c]Status refers to whether or not the initiative was implemented; "Impl" means that it was implemented. [d]Change initiatives were implemented just at the end of the project (month 8).

system to keep track of management feedback to each employee each week. Employees at K-Union developed a colleague feedback system to develop and align work practices and to improve team relations, including a feedback scheme that employees could use to conduct a feedback session. Four sites implemented *work process initiatives*, i.e. EngWater, K-Union, EngPlumb and SocEco. For example, EngWater implemented an initiative to reduce interruptions that used signs on office doors which indicated availability and entailed improving the internal distribution of tasks and making it legitimate to say no to tasks. EngPlumb implemented four initiatives related to interruptions: (1) rules on how to approach colleagues in open offices; (2) rules on telephone noise and a procedure to transfer calls during demanding periods; (3) coloured do-not-disturb signs to help colleagues determine whether a colleague can be interrupted; and (4) email norms on how quickly emails should be checked and answered. EngPlumb also introduced a workload planning initiative, which included a checklist to clarify expectations between project leaders and employees related to minor tasks, and a weekly meeting between the department manager and project leaders to coordinate the workload of employees. SocEco implemented one interruption initiative but did not implement a do-not-disturb signs initiative. SocEco also implemented a revision to its meeting schedule and structure, focusing on inviting only the necessary participants.

Differences between cases also occurred with regard to the scales of the initiatives, their level of adoption and support for the implementation. The initiatives at EngWater and K-Union tended to be larger and were adopted by more employees than those at EngPlumb and SocEco. For instance, despite putting a great deal of effort into concretizing interruption initiatives at EngPlumb and SocEco, few employees in these cases adopted them, possibly because employees viewed them as violating social interaction norms (e.g. do-not-disturb signs). This suggests that the social meaning of such initiatives was not considered in the implementation process in these cases. EngWater was the only workplace that took the social implications of the interruption initiatives into account (e.g. by discussing their social consequences at staff meetings) and fewer difficulties were encountered. In addition, progress was faster at EngWater and K-Union than at EngPlumb and SocEco. The results so far therefore suggest that the cases could be grouped into high-, medium- and non-implementation groups that differed with regard to the type and extent of initiatives and the speed of implementation. In particular, EngWater and K-Union can be placed in the high-implementation group, EngPlumb and SocEco can be placed in a medium-implementation group, while T-Design and SocSecr can be placed into a non-implementation group.

Further differences between the three groups were found with regard to the support provided during implementation. In the high-implementation group, the qualitative analysis suggested that initiative leaders, who were responsible for initiative implementation, were better than those in the other implementation groups at engaging employees in the implementation process. This is also reflected in the survey results, with employees in the high-implementation group reporting significantly higher involvement in project-related activities than employees in the medium- and non-implementation groups (see Table 2, Row 3; $F = 2.41, p < .05$). Employees in the high-implementation group received support right after the workshop, whereas there was a delay of two months in the medium-implementation cases. This is reflected in the survey results showing that support provided by departmental managers for the intervention was significantly higher in the high-implementation group than in the medium- and non-implementation groups (see Table 2, Row 7; $F = 3.68, p < .05$).

During the implementation of the change initiatives, observational and interview data indicated that initiative leaders and managers in the high-implementation group maintained employee awareness by making initiatives highly visible by producing posters and leaflets. Indeed, employees in the high-implementation group report received information on the intervention to a significantly greater extent than did employees in the medium- and non-implementation groups (see Table 2, Row 8; $F = 5.75, p < .05$). The qualitative data also indicated that support from senior management for the implementation of initiatives was greatest in the high-implementation group. EngWater had a steering group with local union and top management participation and K-Union senior management continued to show an active interest in the project. In contrast, in the medium-implementation group, senior management did not have a comparable level of involvement during this period, and support from senior management was significantly lower in this group (see Table 2, Row 6; $F = 12.84$, $p < .01$). Overall, our analysis suggests that there were systematic differences between cases in the type, extent and nature of initiative implementation supporting the portioning of cases into three groups: high-, medium- and non-implementation.

Evaluation of the intervention effects

On the basis of the process analysis and the qualitative results, it might be expected that employees in the high-implementation group would report significantly greater improvements in relational job characteristics than the other two groups, because they were the only workplaces to implement relational initiatives. The results of the multilevel regression (see Table 4) indicate that improvements in relational job characteristics were significantly greater in the high-implementation group with regard to all the relational variables except co-worker support. For example, the level of change in manager relationship quality was significantly higher than in the non-implementation group ($\beta = -.45$, $p < .01$) and the medium-implementation group ($\beta = -.45$, $p < .01$). All the significant changes were at a phenomenologically meaningful level. There were no significant changes in the work process measures: workload and work tempo.

A further expectation was that the implementation of work process and relational initiatives would lead to improvements in employee well-being. We therefore expected that the level of reduction in employee burnout in both the high- and medium-implementation groups would be significantly greater than in the non-implementation group. The change in burnout was significantly higher in the high-implementation group than in the non-implementation group ($\beta = .23$, $p < .01$) but not significantly different from the medium-implementation group ($\beta = .10$, *n.s.*).

Discussion

The aims of this paper were to extend our understanding of how OL-OH initiatives can benefit knowledge workers and to shed further light on the implementation factors that shape the success of such initiatives in knowledge work jobs. These were examined both qualitatively and quantitatively. The paper makes a number of contributions to our understanding of these issues. First, our analysis indicates that knowledge workers' key concerns about their job characteristics relate to task ambiguity and uncertainty, as well as task complexity and interdependency. In particular, employees expressed concern about: the difficulties of crafting solutions to ill-defined problems; knowing when a solution was acceptable; the complexity associated with administering, planning and coordinating several projects; and working on tasks that require uninterrupted problem-solving time but which also require knowledge-sharing and coordination with others. Our findings therefore suggest that interventions to bring about positive changes in knowledge work jobs may be most beneficial if focused on reducing task ambiguity and uncertainty. One means of doing this might be to improve the frequency and quality of feedback from managers to reduce uncertainty on task solutions and task progress.

Knowledge work employees did not seek to implement changes that were directly concerned with increasing task control or task variety, which are key components of

Table 4. Results of multilevel regression analysis, showing comparison of change between high-, medium- and non-implementation groups (N = 247).

	Job autonomy	Workload	Work tempo	Manager relationship quality	Leader skill	Leader support	Co-worker support	Burnout
Mean scores at Time 1 and Time 2								
High-implementation	49.4/55.0	61.0/60.0	70.2/66.2	61.8/68.8	52.1/60.6	60.6/67.8	61.4/62.9	35.7/30.7
Medium-implementation	47.9/47.9	57.6/54.2	66.8/63.0	68.1/63.1	59.3/52.9	59.5/56.2	64.0/61.6	32.1/30.4
Non-implementation	54.6/51.1	47.3/46.9	71.7/71.8	66.2/59.9	65.7/58.7	66.4/53.0	57.2/54.8	35.4/40.5
Multilevel analysis								
Comparison with non-implementation group								
Time	.04	.04	.01	.00	–.11	–.12	–.10	.03
High-implementation	–.02	.30**	.01	–.19*	–.42**	–.29**	.17	–.03
Medium-implementation	–.07	.25**	–.07	–.13	–.12	–.14	–.08	–.01
Time × High	.16	–.10	–.20	.52**	.60**	.56**	.16	–.26*
Time × Medium	–.08	–.41	–.13	.00	–.24*	.06	–.01	–.12
Comparison of change with high-implementation group								
Time	.04	.04	.01	.00	–.11	–.12	–.10	.03
Non-implementation	.02	–.27**	–.01	.17*	.37**	.25**	–.14	.03
Medium-implementation	–.06	–.02	–.08	.04	.24**	.11	–.22*	.02
Time × Non-implementation	–.14	.09	.14	–.45**	–.52**	–.49**	–.14	.23*
Time × Medium	–.21	–.05	.04	–.45**	–.76**	–.43**	–.15	.10

Note: A significant interaction effect indicates that change was significantly different from the group in the interaction term to the referent category group. Level 2 control variables are not shown. Missing values reduce N from 311 to 247.
* p < .05, ** p < .01.

traditional job design theory (Humphrey et al., 2007). This may be because the employees already had fairly high levels of task control and variety and because such increases may have led to greater task uncertainty. Indeed, rather than seeking to increase task discretion, a number of the initiatives appeared to be aimed at increasing the level of formalization in response to concerns about task ambiguity and uncertainty (Juillerat, 2010). Such initiatives included the introduction of procedures to improve planning and coordination, to create better meetings, and to regulate social interaction (e.g. to reduce interruptions). Other studies have shown the potential benefits of using formalization to reduce role ambiguity (Organ & Greene, 1981; Podsakoff, Williams, & Todor, 1986), while Stevens, Diedriks, and Philipsen (1992) found a positive relationship between formalized work processes and employee well-being. However, from this study, it is not clear if formalization led to beneficial changes, as changes in formalization were confounded with changes to work processes. It should also be pointed out that employees were not totally unconcerned about having job control. For example, some of the work process initiatives that were suggested by employees could be interpreted as attempts to gain control over their interactions with colleagues and customers in order to carve out time to concentrate on cognitively demanding tasks.

A further contribution of the process evaluation of this study is that it provides insight into the implementation factors that shape the success of the OL-OH initiatives. The study confirms that effective communication, employee acceptance and willingness to adopt a new initiative, together with support from senior management, are important implementation factors in occupational health interventions (Kompier, Geurts, Gründemann, Vink, & Smulders, 1998; Landsbergis & Vivona-Vaughan, 1995; Nielsen et al., 2010). This study shows that support must be given at key points in the intervention process, particularly soon after intervention workshops (when ideas need to be developed further and made workable), and also during the implementation process, to ensure that change initiatives are widely adopted. These findings are in keeping with other studies. However, one particular insight from this study is that established norms concerning social interaction and the differences in meaning that people attached to initiatives were important factors inhibiting the implementation of work process initiatives. This study therefore suggests that the introduction of work process initiatives may require the social meaning and relational implications of workplace changes to be considered during the implementation process and that employees should be made aware that change initiatives may not simply involve bureaucratic changes to rules. Thus, the study confirms lessons from sociotechnical theory related to industrial work, i.e. that social and technical changes are interrelated (Trist, 1978). A further implication of this is that the successful implementation of OL-OH initiatives may require a set of skills that may not be normally possessed by participants who are infrequently engaged in change activities. The handling of such social processes may benefit from the support of a process facilitator similar to the human resources partner in EngWater, who was a facilitator with knowledge about change management and work psychology (Nytrø, Saksvik, Mikkelsen, Bohle, & Quinlan, 2000).

The process evaluation also highlighted the challenges related to implementing work process initiatives by shedding further light on the possible benefits of using formalized rules and procedures in knowledge work jobs. The idea that formalization can be positive in some circumstances has a long tradition (Gouldner, 1954) and is perhaps best expressed by the concept of an enabling bureaucracy (Adler & Borys, 1996; Juillerat, 2010). In enabling bureaucracies, employees are involved in the creation of rules and work procedures and accept formal rules because they are perceived to facilitate work effectiveness. The qualitative process evaluation points to important differences in the implementation of work process initiatives between the high- and medium-implementation groups, related to employee acceptance of the rules and procedures being implemented. In particular, initiative leaders did succeed in convincing the co-workers in the high-implementation group that bureaucracy was enabling. However, the implementation difficulties observed in the study may be related to the exact same central features of knowledge work jobs that they are trying to solve: complexity and uncertainty. Complex processes are difficult to change, and work efficiency in complex knowledge processes requires creativity and knowledge sharing that may be inhibited by too much formalization, which induces scepticism among participants in the change process. Consequently, it is difficult to achieve a fit between the individual and the intervention (Randall & Nielsen, 2012).

Strengths, limitations and future directions

There were a number of strengths to this study: it was longitudinal and used a mixed-methods design combining quantitative and qualitative methods to examine both interventions process and outcomes. The mixed methodology and reliance on data from different sources reduced the likelihood that common method variance would adversely affect the findings. However, one limitation of this study is the lack of a prospective control group, which weakens any conclusion regarding causal relations. Thus, it cannot be stated with certainty that the intervention was the definite cause of change in employee perceptions of the job or in well-being. However, the in-depth process evaluation partially compensates for this (Kompier, Cooper, & Geurts, 2000; Shadish, Cook, & Campbell, 2002) by providing a detailed account, from multiple sources, of how the intervention process led to changes in job characteristics (Kompier et al., 2000). Another limitation is the non-random allocation of employees to groups, such that differences in outcome between groups may be caused by a treatment/selection interaction effect. However, this specific threat seems unlikely as there were no differences between workplaces in intervention activities, or in employee knowledge of the intervention. A further limitation is the relatively small sample size, which means that caution is required when generalizing to other knowledge work jobs. Finally, the short time span of the evaluation means that the study cannot answer whether the changes were sustainable in the long term.

Future studies of occupational health interventions for knowledge workers could focus on whether formalization and the development of an enabling bureaucracy is a valid approach to take. Such studies could also explore the social meanings of formalization and other changes for knowledge workers, as this would provide further information on the applicability of such approaches in this context. Furthermore, future research should also focus on how support can be provided during the implementation of an intervention while developing ideas and action plans in order to complement the support that is typically provided. Finally, future intervention studies could also examine the control that knowledge workers have over when and who they interact with, as this seems to be a central feature of knowledge work jobs.

Conclusion

In conclusion, the findings from this study suggest that occupational health initiatives among knowledge workers should focus on reducing task uncertainty and ambiguity and on increasing an employee's ability to coordinate action with others. The findings suggest that initiatives to improve management and colleague feedback and to formalize rules and procedures regulating task coordination and social interaction can have positive effects on knowledge work job characteristics and on well-being. Adopting strategies typically used in occupational health interventions, such as increasing job discretion and variety, should be carried out in the awareness that they might increase task uncertainty and ambiguity.

A further conclusion of this study is that to improve the likelihood of a successful OL-OH intervention, much effort must be put into the implementation process so as to secure commitment from employees and senior management, to ensure concrete implementation support from persons with change process expertise, to provide information about the intervention to all stakeholders and to ensure that the social meanings and relational implications of change initiatives are widely understood by all involved.

Acknowledgements

The authors thank Vibeke Andersen, Christine Ipsen, Tina Weller and Anders Buch (Technical University of Denmark) and Peter Holdt Christensen (Copenhagen Business School) who participated in designing and conducting the research project.

Funding

The project was supported by the Danish Working Environment Research Fund [grant 24-2006-04].

References

Adler, P. S., & Borys, B. (1996). Two types of bureaucracy: Enabling and coercive. *Administrative Science Quarterly, 41*(1), 61–89.

Alvesson, M. (1993). Organizations as rhetoric: Knowledge-intensive firms and the struggle with ambiguity. *Journal of Management Studies, 30*, 997–1015.

Bambra, C., Egan, M., Thomas, S., Petticrew, M., & Whitehead, M. (2007). The psychosocial and health effects of workplace reorganisation. 2. A systematic review of task restructuring interventions. *Journal of Epidemiology and Community Health, 61*, 1028–1037.

Baumeister, R. F., Vohs, K. D., & Tice, D. M. (2007). The strength model of self-control. *Current Directions in Psychological Science, 16*, 351–355.

Bond, F. W., & Bunce, B. (2001). Job control mediates change in a work reorganization intervention for stress reduction. *Journal of Occupational Health Psychology, 6*, 290–302.

Brinkley, I., Fauth, R., Mahdon, M., & Theodoropoulou, S. (2010). *Is Knowledge Work Better For Us? Knowledge workers*, good work and wellbeing. London: The Work Foundation.

Cordery, J. L. (1999). Job design and the organisational context. In M. Griffin & J. Langham-Fox (Eds.), *Human performance and the workplace* (pp. 5–15). Melbourne: Australian Psychological Society.

Cox, T., Karanika, M., Griffiths, A., & Houdmont, J. (2007). Evaluating organizational-level work stress interventions: Beyond traditional methods. *Work & Stress, 21*, 348–362.

Crabtree, B. F., & Miller, W. L. (1999). *Doing qualitative research*. Thousand Oaks, CA: Sage.

Davenport, T. H. (2005). *Thinking for a living. How to get better performance and results from knowledge workers*. Boston, MA: Harvard Business School Press.

Davenport, T. H., Jarvenpaa, S. L., & Beers, M. C. (1996). Improving knowledge work processes. *Sloan Management Review, 37,* 53–65.

DeFillippi, R., Arthur, M., & Limdsay, V. (2005). *Knowledge at work: Creative collaboration in the global economy.* Boston: Blackwell.

de Lange, A. H., Taris, T. W., Kompier, M. A. J., Houtman, I. L. D., & Bongers, P. M. (2003). The very best of the millennium: Longitudinal research and the Demand-Control(-Support) model. *Journal of Occupational Health Psychology, 8,* 282–305.

Demerouti, E., Bakker, A. B., Nachreiner, F., & Schaufeli, W. B. (2001). The job demands-resources model of burnout. *Journal of Applied Psychology, 86,* 499–512.

Drucker, P. F. (1993). *Post-capitalist society.* Oxford: Butterworth- Heinemann.

Egan, M., Bambra, C., Petticrew, M., & Whitehead, M. (2009). Reviewing evidence on complex social interventions: Appraising implementation in systematic reviews of the health effects of organizational-level workplace interventions. *Journal of Epidemiology and Community Heaith, 63,* 4–11.

Egan, M., Bambra, C., Thomas, S., Petticrew, M., Whitehead, M., & Thomson, H. (2007). The psychosocial and health effects of workplace reorganisation. 1. A systematic review of organisational-level interventions that aim to increase employee control. *Journal of Epidemiology and Community Health, 61,* 945–954.

Gardner, D. G., & Cummings, L. L. (1988). Activation theory and job design - Review and reconceptualization. *Research in Organizational Behavior, 10,* 81–122.

Gibbs, G. (2009). *Analyzing qualitative data.* London: Sage.

Gouldner, A. W. (1954). *Patterns of industrial bureaucracy.* New York, NY: Free Press.

Grant, A. M., & Parker, S. K. (2009). Redesigning work design theories: The rise of relational and proactive perspectives. *Academy of Management Annals, 3,* 317–375.

Grönlund, A. (2007). Employee control in the era of flexibility: A stress buffer or a stress amplifier? *European Societies, 9,* 409–428.

Guest, G., MacQueen, K. M., & Namey, E. E. (2012). *Applied Thematic Analysis.* London: Sage.

Holman, D. J., Axtell, C. M., Sprigg, C. A., Totterdell, P., & Wall, T. D. (2010). The mediating role of job characteristics in job redesign interventions: A serendipitous quasi-experiment. *Journal of Organizational Behavior, 31,* 84–105.

Humphrey, S. E., Nahrgang, J. D., & Morgeson, F. P. (2007). Integrating motivational, social, and contextual work design features: A meta-analytic summary and theoretical extension of the work design literature. *Journal of Applied Psychology, 92,* 1332–1356.

Juillerat, T. L. (2010). Friends, not foes?: Work design and formalization in the modern work context. *Journal of Organizational Behavior, 31,* 216–239.

Karasek, R. A., & Theorell, T. (1990). *Healthy work - Stress, productivity, and the reconstruction of working life.* New York, NY: Basic Books.

Kinman, G., & Jones, F. (2008). Effort-reward imbalance, over-commitment and work-life conflict: Testing an expanded model. *Journal of Managerial Psychology, 23,* 236–251.

Kompier, M. A. J., Cooper, C. L., & Geurts, S. A. E. (2000). A multiple case study approach to work stress prevention in Europe. *European Journal of Work and Organizational Psychology, 9,* 371–400.

Kompier, M. A. J., Geurts, S. A. E., Grundemann, R. W. M., Vink, P., & Smulders, P. G. W. (1998). Cases in stress prevention: The success of a participative and stepwise approach. *Stress Medicine, 14,* 155–168.

Kristensen, T. S., Hannerz, H., Hogh, A., & Borg, V. (2005). The Copenhagen Psychosocial Questionnaire - a tool for the assessment and improvement of the psychosocial work environment. *Scandinavian Journal of Work Environment & Health, 31,* 438–449.

Landsbergis, P. A., & Vivona-Vaughan, E. (1995). Evaluation of an occupational stress intervention in a public agency. *Journal of Organizational Behavior, 16*(1), 29–48.

McClenahan, C. A., Giles, M. L., & Mallett, J. (2007). The importance of context specificity in work stress research: A test of the Demand-Control-Support model in academics. *Work & Stress, 21,* 85–95.

McGrath, J. E. (1976). Stress and behavior in organizations. In *Handbook of industrial and organizational psychology* (pp. 1351–1395). Chicago, IL: Rand-McNally.

Nastasi, B. K., Hitchcock, J., Sarkar, S., Burkholder, G., Varjas, K., & Jayasena, A. (2007). Mixed methods in intervention research. *Journal of Mixed Methods Research, 1,* 164–182.

Nielsen, K., & Abildgaard, J. S. (2013). Organizational interventions: A research-based framework for the evaluation of both process and effects. *Work & Stress, 27*, 278–297.

Nielsen, K., Randall, R., & Albertsen, K. (2007). Participants' appraisals of process issues and the effects of stress management interventions. *Journal of Organizational Behavior, 28*, 793–810.

Nielsen, K., Randall, R., Holten, A.-L., & Rial González, E. (2010). Conducting organizational-level occupational health interventions: What works? *Work & Stress, 24*, 234–259.

Nielsen, K., Taris, T. W., & Cox, T. (2010). The future of organizational interventions: Addressing the challenges of today's organizations. *Work & Stress, 24*, 219–233.

NVivo (8.0) [computer software]. Retrieved from http://www.qsrinternational.com/

Nytrø, K., Saksvik, P. Ø., Mikkelsen, A., Bohle, P., & Quinlan, M. (2000). An appraisal of key factors in the implementation of occupational stress interventions. *Work & Stress, 14*, 213–225.

Organ, D. W., & Greene, C. N. (1981). The effects of formalization on professional involvement: A compensatory process approach. *Administrative Science Quarterly, 26*, 237–252.

Pejtersen, J. H., Bjørner, J. B., & Hasle, P. (2010). Determining minimally important score differences in scales of the Copenhagen Psychosocial Questionnaire. *Scandinavian Journal of Public Health, 38*(3 Suppl), 33–41.

Podsakoff, P. M., Williams, L. J., & Todor, W. D. (1986). Effects of organizational formalization on alienation among professionals and nonprofessionals. *The Academy of Management Journal, 29*, 820–831.

Quené, H., & van den Bergh, H. (2004). On multi-level modeling of data from repeated measures designs: a tutorial. *Speech Communication, 43*(1–2), 103–121.

Randall, R., & Nielsen, K. (2012). Does the intervention fit? An explanatory model of intervention success and failure in complex organizational environments. In C. Biron, M. Karanika-Murray, & C. L. Cooper (Eds.), *Improving organizational interventions on stress and well-being: Addressing process and context* (pp. 120–134). London: Psychology Press.

Randall, R., Nielsen, K., & Tvedt, S. D. (2009). The development of five scales to measure employees' appraisals of organizational-level stress management interventions. *Work & Stress, 23*(1), 1–23.

Raudenbush, S., Bryk, A., Cheong, Y. K., & Congdon, R. (1999). *HLM 5: Hierarchical linear and non-linear modelling.* Lincolnwood, IL: Scientific Software International.

Rugulies, R., Martin, M. H. T., Garde, A. H., Persson, R., & Albertsen, K. (2012). Deadlines at work and sleep quality. Cross-sectional and longitudinal findings among Danish knowledge workers. *American Journal of Industrial Medicine, 55*, 260–269.

Semmer, N. K. (2006). Job stress interventions and the organization of work. *Scandinavian Journal of Work Environment & Health, 32*, 515–527.

Shadish, W. R., & Cook, T. D. (1999). Comment-Design rules: More steps toward a complete theory of quasi-experimentation. *Statistical Science, 14*, 294–300.

Shadish, W. R., Cook, T. D., & Campbell, D. T. (2002). *Experimental and quasi-experimental designs for generalized causal inference.* Boston, MA: Houghton Mifflin.

Stevens, F., Diederiks, J., & Philipsen, H. (1992). Physician satisfaction, professional characteristics, and behavior formalization in hospitals. *Social Science and Medicine, 35*, 295–303.

Trist, E. L. (1978). On socio-technical systems. In W. Passmore & J. Sherwood (Eds.), *Sociotechnical systems: A sourcebook.* (pp. 43–58). San Diego, CA: University Associates

Xie, J. L., & Johns, G. (1995). Job scope and stress - Can job scope be too high. *Academy of Management Journal, 38*, 1288–1309.

Should I stay or should I go? Examining longitudinal relations among job resources and work engagement for stayers versus movers

Annet H. de Lange[a], Hans De Witte[b] and Guy Notelaers[b,c]

[a]Department of Social and Organizational Psychology, University of Groningen, The Netherlands; [b]Research Group Work, Organizational and Personnel Psychology (WOPP), Department of Psychology, Katholieke Universiteit Leuven, Belgium; [c]Department of Psychosocial Science, Faculty of Psychology, University of Bergen, Norway

This two-wave (16-month lag) Belgian panel study is one of the first to test theory-driven hypotheses on the relations between job resources, work engagement, and actual turnover across time. The study focuses on three groups: stayers, workers who have obtained promotions ("promotion makers"), and external job movers. In line with the Job Demands-Resources model, we hypothesized normal cross-lagged effects of job resources on work engagement for stayers. Based on broaden-and-build theory, a reversed causal effect of work engagement on job resources was predicted for the job changers. Additionally, we examined whether the changes in the job change groups matched the refuge hypothesis (that less engaged workers change to jobs providing more resources) or the positive gain hypothesis (that engaged workers get promoted to jobs having even more resources). The results partially supported our hypotheses. We found that low work engagement, low job autonomy, and low departmental resources predicted actual transfer to another company. Furthermore, for stayers we found positive effects of job autonomy on work engagement, but also reversed causal effects. For external movers and promotion makers the expected reversed causal effects of work engagement were found. The across time mean changes support the positive gain hypothesis for promotion makers, and the refuge hypothesis for external movers.

Introduction

In view of an increasing shortfall of qualified and competent workers, practitioners as well as scholars have realized that in order to survive in the dynamic global economy it is crucial to retain and motivate one's personnel (Martin, 2005; Ployhart, 2006). It has become increasingly important to examine the conditions and processes that contribute to the optimal functioning and happiness of people (Gable & Haidt, 2005; Warr, 2007). In line with this "positive psychology" movement of focusing on human strengths at work rather than on weaknesses and ill-health (Cooper, 2005; Gable & Haidt, 2005), we wanted to examine the causal nature of the relations among job resources and work engagement in a longitudinal perspective. As earlier organizational research in this area has minimized the role of worker behaviour in changing his or her own work environment, we will also pay attention to the role of employees in shaping their own work environment by examining the differences between stayers versus job changers (Wrzesniewski & Dutton, 2001).

Work engagement refers to a positive affective-motivational state of fulfillment that is characterized by vigour, dedication, and absorption (Schaufeli, Salanova, González-Romá, & Bakker, 2002). In the current study we will focus on the two core dimensions of engagement (Bakker, Schaufeli, Leiter, & Taris, 2008; González-Romá, Schaufeli, Bakker, & Lloret, 2006): vigour (i.e., high level of energy and mental resilience while working) and dedication (i.e., a strong involvement in one's work and feelings of enthusiasm, significance, a sense of pride and inspiration). Work engagement is a crucial factor in sustaining well-being and productivity of workers as it has been linked to performance and creativity as well as to health (Bakker, 2008). According to the job demands-resources (JD-R) model (Bakker & Demerouti, 2007; Demerouti, Bakker, Nachreiner, & Schaufeli, 2001), *job resources* play a vital role in the development of work engagement, and refer to physical, social, or organizational aspects of the job that are functional in obtaining work goals, reducing job demands, and providing opportunities for personal growth and learning.

Job resources can play in this context either an intrinsic motivational role through increasing employees' growth, learning and development, or an extrinsic motivational role in achieving work goals (Bakker, 2008). For example, the team-related resource "social support" may fulfil the basic human need of wanting to relate to others, whereas the task-related resource "task autonomy" may fulfil needs for autonomy and competence (Deci & Ryan, 1985; Ryan & Frederick, 1997; Van den Broeck, Vansteenkiste, De Witte, & Lens, 2008). According to conservation of resources (COR) theory (Halbesleben, 2006; Hobfoll, 1985), job resources like social support or support provided at the departmental level play an important role in reinforcing positive images of oneself, and in fostering positive work outcomes like work engagement (Demerouti et al., 2001). Social support or job autonomy may also play an extrinsic motivational role in better achieving work goals (Bakker, 2008).

As the JD-R model and the concept of work engagement are relatively new, an overview of earlier studies focusing on the relation between job resources and work engagement is still missing. We therefore conducted a literature review of earlier published studies and found 16 empirical studies that reported strong positive relations (e.g., high standardized betas or correlations) between job resources and work engagement across homogeneous (69%) as well as heterogenous (31%) samples. (See marked references in reference section; a table with more detailed information about the selected studies can be obtained from the first author.) The significant predictive job resources that were included varied from task-related resources (like job control or autonomy), to social or team-related resources (like social support) and to organizational-level resources (like social climate or information; cf. Bakker, Hakanen, Demerouti, & Xanthopoulou, 2007; Salanova, Agut, & Peiró, 2005; Xanthopoulou, Bakker, Demerouti, & Schaufeli, 2007). In all reviewed studies, work engagement was measured using the Utrecht Work Engagement Scale (Schaufeli & Bakker, in press; Schaufeli & Bakker, 2008), presenting relatively high psychometric quality across all studies. However, there were a number of unresolved issues, related to the design used and tested causal directions of the relations, that we would like to address in the present two-wave study.

Paucity of longitudinal field studies

Only three of the 16 selected studies (19%) used a longitudinal design (e.g., two measurements or more across time). First, Llorens, Schaufeli, Bakker, and Salanova (2007) found significant reciprocal relations between task resources (time and method control) and engagement (mediated by efficacy beliefs) in a longitudinal study among 110 university students. Unfortunately, as only university students were examined in a laboratory setting it is difficult to generalize these results to the working population. The longitudinal study of Mauno, Kinnunen, and Ruokolainen (2007) is based on a sample of workers in a real life context. They reported positive cross-lagged relations between job resources (job control, organization-based self-esteem, and management quality) and work engagement using a sample of Finnish public health employees, and a time-lag of two years. Finally, Sonnentag (2003) examined a sample of workers of six different public service organizations in a diary study, and found significant positive effects of method control on work engagement.

Our literature review also showed that whereas a wide range of job resources has been examined in cross-sectional studies, only a few different types of job resources have been examined in the longitudinal studies. More explicit longitudinal tests with different types of job resources, and testing respondents in their actual work setting, are needed. In this study we will therefore examine a task-related resource (autonomy), team-related resources (social support from colleagues and social support from supervisors), as well as departmental resources (e.g., enough staff, good organization of department), among a heterogeneous group of workers.

Normal, reversed, or reciprocal causation?

Another limitation of the selected studies is their uni-directional view on the relations between job resources and work engagement. Structural models such as the JD-R model focus on specific aspects of the complex psychosocial work environment to explain how individuals perceive and react to their job, and postulate the relations between job resources and work engagement as uni-directional. In other words, these models hypothesize that job resources as measured at one point in time will influence work engagement at a later point in time (denoted as "normal" causal relationships in the remainder of this study), but not vice versa. In line with this idea, a large majority of the selected studies (94%) examined only the normal causal effects of job resources on work engagement. However, increasingly, longitudinal research suggests that the uni-directional view of work and mental health conveyed in job stress models like the JD-R model may be too narrow (Bakker & Demerouti, 2007; De Lange, Taris, Kompier, Houtman, & Bongers, 2004; De Lange, Taris, Kompier, Houtman, & Bongers, 2005; Frese, Garst, & Fay, 2007; Hakanen, Schaufeli, & Ahola, 2008).

The associations between job resources and work engagement may be explained by *reversed* causal relationships (in which Time 1 engagement influences [the evaluation of] Time 2 job resources) or *reciprocal* (bi-directional) relationships in which job resources and work engagement mutually influence each other (Zapf, Dormann, & Frese, 1996). Of our reviewed studies, only the study of Llorens et al. (2007) tested for normal, reversed, and reciprocal effects of engagement, and reported significant reciprocal effects. They showed that task resources, through enhancing one's efficacy beliefs, can increase work engagement, but that work engagement, in turn, can positively influence efficacy beliefs and task resources across time. This study revealed that employees can be regarded as active shapers or job crafters of their work environment, rather than as passive receivers only (cf. Taris, Bok, & Caljé, 1998; Wrzesniewski & Dutton, 2001). Nonetheless, the question remains why reversed effects of work engagement occur and which possible mechanisms may explain normal versus reversed effects among job resources and work engagement.

Differentiating stayers from movers

In line with Kasl and Jones (2003), we think that especially the baseline pre-change data and cross-lagged changes found for stayers versus movers can provide more information about normal versus reversed cause-and-effect relationships. We will therefore examine the nature and form of the cross-lagged relations between job resources and work engagement across stayers (workers who remain in the same work environment) versus self-determined movers (workers who have obtained promotions, labelled as promotion makers, or transferred to a different company, labelled as external movers). According to a meta-analysis of Griffeth, Hom, and Gaertner (2000), few resources (e.g., limited participation and instrumental communication) and low psychological well-being (e.g., job dissatisfaction) are significant predictors of personnel turnover. Similarly, Schaufeli, Taris, Le Blanc, Peeters, Bakker, and De Jonge (2001) found in their interview study that low work engagement can be a significant predictor of turnover, and Schaufeli and Bakker (2004) found in their multi-sample study that work engagement was related negatively to turnover intention. However, work engagement and job resources have never been examined in relation to actual turnover across time. We therefore want to examine whether the baseline level of work engagement as well as job resources can predict whether individuals will stay in the same work environment or actively shape their environment through achieving promotion or choosing to transfer to another company. We therefore tested the following hypotheses:

> *Hypothesis 1a:* In line with the meta-analysis of Griffeth et al. (2000), we expect that low work engagement and limited job resources will be predictive for changing to another company. As these workers are confronted with a less resourceful job, they will be more motivated to look for better ones.

> *Hypothesis 1b:* On the other hand, resourceful jobs will not inspire transferance to another company. Hence, we expect that high work engagement and many job resources will be predictive for staying in the same job or obtaining a promotion.

In order to formulate more theory-driven hypotheses for normal versus reversed effects among these different exposure groups, we will refer to broaden-and-build principles of positive emotions (cf. Fredrickson, 2001) as well as the environmental change mechanisms recently suggested by De Lange, Taris, Kompier, Houtman, and Bongers (2005).

Normal causation among stayers

In line with the broaden-and-build theory of positive emotions (Fredrickson, 2001), we argue that positive emotions, like work engagement, have the capacity to broaden one's thought-action repertoires and to increase or build more job resources. Through widening one's possible thoughts and actions, engaged workers will be better at mobilizing their job resources or in utilizing promotion opportunities, which might increase their capacities for emotion regulation (Gross, 1998; Halbesleben, 2006; Hobfoll, 2001; Salanova, Bakker, & Llorens, 2006). As stayers have not selected different work situations or actively crafted their current work situation to regulate their emotions, we expect to find less reversed effects of their work engagement across time compared to the job change groups. Hence:

Hypothesis 2: We expect normal causal effects of job resources in predicting work engagement across time for the group of stayers.

Positive reversed causation among promotion makers

Following Fredrickson's (2001) broaden-and-build theory of positive emotions, we expect to find reversed causal effects for the job changers. However, as we differentiate two groups of job changers (promotion makers and external movers), the direction of the reversed effects can be either positive or negative. De Lange et al. (2005) distinguish two different environmental change mechanisms that can be used to theorize about the positive as well as negative reversed effects of work engagement among promotion makers and external movers. These mechanisms include: (1) internal job changes, in which, for example, the *increased* work engagement of a worker results in self-determined *positive* changes of the current job (worker seeks new challenges); or (2) external job changes due to job transfer. For example, the increased work engagement allows for career transitions towards new challenging or more resourceful work environments (Frese et al., 2007; Wrzesniewski & Dutton, 2001). In this *upward selection* process or positive gain spiral hypothesis, relatively more engaged workers get *promoted* to more-challenging jobs (with challenging tasks, but also more job control or departmental resources; Ganster & Schabroeck, 1991, p. 263). In line with this positive gain spiral hypothesis, we expect that:

> *Hypothesis 3a*: Positive reversed effects will be found for the promotion makers (e.g., work engagement will predict more job resources across time); and
> *Hypothesis 3b*: A higher overall level of job resources as well as work engagement will be found after their promotion.

Negative reversed causation among external movers

For the *external movers*, the situation may be more complex. The external movers may reveal similar positive effects as the promotion makers when they are highly engaged. However, as earlier research has indicated that low psychological well-being is often the reason to transfer to another company (Griffeth et al., 2000; Schaufeli & Bakker, 2004; Schaufeli et al., 2001), we expect to find external movers to be relatively less engaged (see *Hypothesis 1a*). An explanation for positive across-time changes among less engaged workers is the "refuge hypothesis." According to this hypothesis, and in line with assumptions of COR-theory (Hobfoll, 2001), *less engaged* workers will organize their jobs/positions differently or look for "refuge" in new jobs to create more resourceful work environments (De Lange et al., 2005; Garst, Frese, & Molenaar, 2000). An explanation for reversed effects of low work engagement is the so-called "drift mechanism" (Frese, 1985; Zapf et al., 1996). Accordingly, workers with low work engagement will be less successful in changing their situation and "drift" off to worse jobs (resulting in a negative loss spiral). This downward selection process (Ettner & Grzywacz, 2001) can be understood as a derivative of the familiar healthy worker effect (Marmot & Madge, 1987), namely, the assumption that only healthy and engaged workers are able to retain a certain job implies that less engaged workers are *un*able to do so. Unfortunately, no study to date has validated these different mechanisms for reversed effects of work engagement among different job change groups, and we will therefore provide a first test of these potential reversed effects of work engagement.

We will employ a positive perspective on the role of workers in changing their environment and expect, in line with the aforementioned "refuge hypothesis" (De Lange et al., 2005; Garst et al., 2000), that:

> *Hypothesis 4a*: Negative reversed effects will be found for the external movers (e.g., low work engagement will predict more job resources across time); and
>
> *Hypothesis 4b*: The external movers will show a higher overall level of job resources as well as work engagement after the external move.

Method

Participants and procedure

Study design

To test our hypotheses, a complete two-wave panel study was conducted, with a time lag of approximately 16 months. The follow-up survey (T2) was planned originally for 12 months after T1. Due to practical constraints, however, this was likely to be impossible, and the time lag had to be extended to 16 months. Note that several researchers (e.g., Dormann & Zapf, 2002; Mauno et al., 2007) showed that even a time lag of two years can be adequate to demonstrate a relationship between job characteristics and psychological outcomes. The first survey was posted at the end of 2003 on a website of a Belgian HR-magazine. In total, 4175 workers responded to the first survey. All of them received an email inviting them to participate in the second wave of this web survey (May 2005). In total, 1670 participants responded (response rate = 40%). This response rate is comparable to those registered in other studies (Mauno, Kinnunen, Mäkikangas, & Nätti, 2005). After excluding unemployed respondents and workers who reported no self-determined changes due to organizational changes and restructuring, the selected sample size equalled 871 respondents.

Drop-out

A comparison between the respondents of the second wave and those who dropped out after wave 1 did not reveal important differences between the groups, suggesting that selection on core variables was limited or non-existent (for more information, see De Cuyper, Notelaers, & De Witte, in press). Those who participated in the second wave of the survey were compared to those who dropped out on all relevant variables. The drop out group scored slightly lower on most items, which suggests a limited selection effect (the drop out group scored lower than the participants on, for example, support from colleagues scores respectively 3.01 versus 3.07 on a 5-point scale, $p < .001$) and support from supervisors (scores respectively 2.82 versus 2.87 on a 5-point scale, $p < .001$). The drop out group was also younger than the participants at T1 (respectively 34.3 versus 36.4 years of age, $p < .01$). It seems unlikely that these differences significantly distorted our results.

Sample

The mean age of our respondents was 36.2 years ($SD = 10.0$) and mean job tenure was 6.4 years ($SD = 7.6$). Slightly more female (53.5%) compared to male (45.6%) workers participated. About 12% worked part-time, and 13% were employed with a temporary contract. All sectors (e.g., industry and service) were represented. Respondents were dominantly working in the private sector (68.5%), with 27.7% working in the public sector and 3.2% working as self-employed. The distribution of the educational level showed that highly educated workers were overrepresented. The level of education was low for 7.3%, moderate for 21.6% (secondary education), whereas 70.7% completed some form of higher education (43.5% non-university and 27.2% university). Most respondents were "routine non-manual employees" (34.7%) or "professionals, administrators, and managers" (57.5%).

Job status

The analysis of changes between wave 1 and 2 shows that 69.2% ($N = 603$) of the respondents remained in the same job (experienced no change in employer, supervisor, work location, or colleagues; labelled as "stayers"), 14.1% ($N = 123$) obtained a promotion or better job with the same employer ("promotion makers"), and 16.6% ($N = 145$) obtained a new job with a different employer (labelled as "external movers"). All changes referred to the period since the first wave was conducted (i.e., to the previous 16 months).

Measures

Job autonomy was measured by a 3-item job autonomy scale (e.g., "I can take many decisions in my job autonomously"; 1 = "totally disagree," 7 = "totally agree"). The items were derived from the Short-Inventory on Stress and Well-being (S-ISW; Vander Elst, Eertmans, Taeymans, & De Witte, 2008). The reliability (Cronbach's alpha) of the job autonomy scale was on Time 1 = .94 and Time 2 = .82.

Social support was measured with three items from the social support from colleagues scale (e.g., "Can you count on your colleagues when work gets difficult?"; 1 = "never," 4 = "always"), and a 3-item support from supervisors scale (e.g., "Do you feel valued by your direct supervisor at work?"; 1 = "never," 4 = "always"). Both were derived from the Questionnaire on the Experience and Evaluation of Work (van Veldhoven & Meijman, 1994). The reliabilities (Cronbach's alpha) of the social support from colleagues scales were Time 1 = .75 and Time 2 = .74. For social support from supervisors, these alpha's were Time 1 = .87 and Time 2 = .86.

Departmental resources was measured by a 4-item scale, tapping experienced resources at the unit/departmental level (e.g., "The work is well organized in my unit/department," "There are enough staff/personnel in my unit/department to perform well"; 1 = "totally disagree," 7 = "totally agree"). The questions were derived from the S-ISW (Vander Elst et al., 2008). The reliability (Cronbach's alpha) of the scale was at Time 1 = .77 and Time 2 = .78.

Work engagement was measured with a 6-item version of the Utrecht Work Engagement Scale (UWES; Schaufeli & Bakker, 2004), measuring the core concepts of vigour (e.g., "At my work, I feel bursting with energy"), and dedication (e.g., "My job inspires me") (Bakker et al., 2008; González-Romá et al., 2006). Participants could respond using a 7-point scale (0 = "never," 6 = "always"). The scores on both scales were summed to form one overall score for work engagement. The reliability (Cronbach's alpha) of the work engagement scale was alpha T1 = .94, and T2 = .95.

Covariates. As many studies have already shown that it is important to control for covariates like demographics and indicators of socio economic status (cf. Bakker, Demerouti, & Schaufeli, 2005; Bakker et al., 2007), we controlled for the influence of age, gender, worker position, and years of experience.

Statistical analysis

Correlational analyses were conducted to obtain more basic insight into the data, and descriptive discriminant analysis was used to examine whether the baseline levels of work engagement and job resource scores were predictive of job status (staying, promotion making, or external movers) (Stevens, 1996). We employed two common methods for interpreting discriminant functions: we examined the standardized coefficients as well as the discriminant function-variable correlations. The largest coefficients or correlations are used for interpretation (Stevens, 1996). Age, gender, worker position, and years of experience were included as control variables in these and all following analyses.

Further, structural equation modelling (SEM) analysis (Jöreskog & Sörbom, 1993) was used to test and compare simultaneously various competing models for the relationships between job resources and work engagement across time among stayers, promotion makers, and external movers. We performed a comparative analysis in which the fit of several competing models was assessed to determine which model fitted the data best (Kelloway, 1998). All results presented below are based on the standardized results. The following tests were used to evaluate our models: the chi-square difference test, the goodness-of–fit index (GFI), the root-mean square error of approximation (RMSEA), and the standardized root mean square residual (SRMR). Levels of .90 or better for GFI levels, and .05 or lower for RMSEA and SRMR indicate that the models fit the data reasonably well (Byrne, 2002).

Considering the problems caused by estimating all observed items and latent variables (insufficient power and under-identification: Bentler & Chou, 1987; Schumacker & Lomax, 1996), we assumed the observed and latent variables to be identical. We calculated the sum scores based upon the indicators of the latent construct. Following the two-step approach proposed by James, Mulaik, and Brett (1982), we first tested the measurement models for each of the variables before fitting the structural models. These analyses showed that the factor structures of the research variables were consistent across time. Structural equation analyses showed that imposing the measurement structure simultaneously on the data at Time 1 and Time 2 is associated with an acceptable fitting model ($\chi^2(601) = 2239.14$; RMSEA $= .05$, RMR $= 0.04$, GFI $= .90$).

Competing structural models

To examine the causal relationships between the job resources and work engagement, we tested a baseline model versus several competing nested models. More specifically, these models were:

1. *Baseline or stability model* (M_1): Includes temporal stabilities and synchronous (i.e., within-wave) effects of variables over time and controls for the influence of covariates (age, gender, job tenure and worker position). This model is used as the reference model.
2. *Normal causation model* (M_2): This model resembles M_1, but includes additional cross-lagged structural paths from the Time 1 job resources to Time 2 work engagement.
3. *Reversed causation model* (M_3): This models resembles M_1, but is extended with cross-lagged structural paths from Time 1 work engagement to Time 2 job resources.
4. *Reciprocal causation model* (M_4): This model resembles M_1, but includes additional reciprocal cross-lagged structural paths from job resources to work engagement and vice versa (i.e., the normal paths included in model M_2 as well as the reversed paths included in model M_3).

To examine Hypotheses 2, 3a, and 4a, we performed multiple-group analyses and compared the aforementioned nested models simultaneously for all job status groups by means of the chi-square difference test (Jöreskog & Sorbom, 1993). A Manova with repeated measures was used to further examine the across-time changes and differences in the job change groups (Hypotheses 3b–4b).

Results

Descriptive statistics

Tables 1 and 2 present the correlations among the variables under study for the total group of workers, the stayers, promotion makers, and external movers separately. As regards the across-time stability of the variables, the correlations for the group of stayers were (as was to be expected) higher compared with the promotion makers, and especially the external movers. The Time 1–Time 2 test–retest correlations ranged from .13 (for social support supervisor among the external movers) to .71 (for work engagement among the stayers).

Inferential statistics

According to Hypotheses 1a and b, we expected that low work engagement and limited job resources would be predictive for changing to another company, and that high work engagement and job resources would be predictive for staying in the same job or obtaining a promotion. Table 3 presents the results of our discriminant analysis examining the influence of the job resources and work engagement on respondents' job status. The results reveal that it is primarily departmental resources, job autonomy and work engagement that distinguish the external movers from the stayers and promotion makers. More specifically, low work engagement, few departmental resources as well as low job autonomy are significant predictors of changing to another company. The function at group centroids shows that these variables are positive (but less strong) predictors for the stayers and promotion makers (supporting Hypothesis 1a, and providing partial support for Hypothesis 1b).

According to Hypotheses 2, 3a, and 4a, we expected normal cross-lagged effects for stayers, positive reversed cross-lagged effects for promotion makers, and negative reversed cross-lagged effects for external movers. To test these hypotheses, we compared the fit of the baseline or stability model, the normal causation, reversed causation, and the reciprocal model using multi-group SEM-analyses. Table 4 presents the fit indices and chi-square difference tests of these analyses, revealing that the reciprocal model fits better to the data for all groups compared to the stability (M_4 versus M_1: $\Delta\chi^2(14) = 44.28$, $p < .01$), and the normal causation model (M_4 versus M_2: $\Delta\chi^2(12) = 24.88$, $p < .05$). However, the fit of the reciprocal model was not significantly better than the reversed causation model (M_4 versus M_2: $\Delta\chi^2(12) = 17.88$, $p > .05$).

After examining the standardized cross-lagged effects (procedure recommended by Jöreskog & Sörbom, 1993) among the stayers, we only found a significant normal effect of Time 1 job autonomy on Time 2 work engagement ($\beta = .08$, $p < .01$), but also significant reversed effects of Time 1 work engagement on Time 2 colleague support ($\beta = .04$, $p < .01$) and supervisor support ($\beta = .05$, $p < .01$). Note that the effects are small, but in the expected direction. Among the promotion makers we found the predicted positive reversed effects of Time 1 work engagement on Time 2 job autonomy ($\beta = .20$, $p < .01$), and on Time 2 departmental resources ($\beta = .20$, $p < .01$). For the external movers only a significant negative reversed effect was found of Time 1 work engagement on Time 2 colleague support

Table 1. Correlations between research variables for all groups (N = 871 after listwise deletion) are presented in upper diagonal, results of stayers (N = 603 after listwise deletion) in lower diagonal.

Variables	1	2	3	4	5	6	7	8	9	10	11	12	13	14
Time 1														
1. Age	–	-.28	.60	.15	.14	-.00	.04	.09	.14	.13	-.01	.05	.11	.13
2. Gender[a]	-.19	–	-.07	-.12	-.06	.05	.03	.03	.03	-.08	.04	-.01	.04	.03
3. Job tenure	.61	-.10	–	-.00	.05	-.03	-.06	.04	.02	.08	-.00	-.01	.05	.04
4. Worker position[a]	.10	-.08	-.04	–	.35	.06	.10	.12	.23	.24	.01	.04	.06	.11
5. Autonomy	.10	-.01	.01	.36	–	.40	.57	.60	.69	.60	.24	.33	.35	.44
6. Support colleague	-.01	.07	-.05	.05	.39	–	.55	.46	.44	.24	.52	.34	.26	.27
7. Support supervisor	.01	.03	-.10	.09	.57	.56	–	.60	.55	.31	.32	.49	.33	.36
8. Departmental resources	.06	.08	-.03	.12	.56	.46	.60	–	.50	.38	.30	.36	.55	.35
9. Work engagement	.09	.08	-.02	.22	.67	.45	.54	.49	–	.40	.26	.29	.28	.59
Time 2														
10. Autonomy	.16	-.04	.09	.28	.70	.26	.36	.43	.47	–	.42	.54	.57	.68
11. Support colleague	.01	-.01	.02	.03	.33	.60	.37	.34	.35	.42	–	.53	.46	.45
12. Support supervisor	.09	.03	.03	.05	.41	.39	.61	.46	.37	.50	.54	–	.56	.51
13. Departmental resources	.15	.02	.06	.10	.42	.29	.39	.67	.33	.58	.46	.55	–	.53
14. Work engagement	.15	.12	.05	.14	.55	.33	.41	.41	.71	.67	.46	.49	.51	–

Note: $r \geq (-).08$ are significant at the .05 level; [a]. Gender: 1 = female, 2 = male;
Worker position: 1 = blue collar work, 2 = lower level white collar work, 3 = self-employed, 4 = job in care or education (e.g., nurse or teacher), 5 = middle level white collar, professional or "free" profession, 6 = higher level white collar worker, management.

Table 2. Correlations between research variables for external movers ($N = 145$ after listwise deletion) are presented in the upper diagonal, and results promotion makers ($N = 123$ after listwise deletion) in the lower diagonal.

	Variables	1	2	3	4	5	6	7	8	9	10	11	12	13	14
	Time 1														
1	Age	–	-.07	.50	.31	.13	-.04	.00	-.10	.23	.00	-.17	-.07	.14	.11
2	Gender[a]	-.15	–	.15	-.20	-.14	.04	-.01	-.02	-.12	-.09	.04	-.04	.12	.01
3	Job tenure	.53	-.04	–	.15	.08	-.04	-.06	.03	.13	.11	-.08	-.06	-.03	.16
4	Worker position[a]	.14	-.19	-.07	–	.32	.04	.10	.03	.25	.16	-.10	.06	-.08	.06
5	Autonomy	.14	-.09	-.05	.29	–	.34	.51	.57	.71	.25	-.03	.07	.10	.16
6	Support colleague	-.07	.02	-.08	.08	.44	–	.54	.45	.39	.10	.28	.19	.08	.09
7	Support supervisor	.05	.12	-.15	.01	.56	.50	–	.61	.52	.06	.18	.13	.08	.19
8	Departmental resources	.15	-.03	.02	.06	.62	.45	.52	–	.44	.20	.20	.19	.22	.21
9	Work engagement	.11	.05	-.08	.19	.67	.42	.50	.52	–	.09	-.06	-.02	.02	.20
	Time 2														
10	Autonomy	.08	-.20	-.06	.08	.56	.29	.36	.43	.50	–	.40	.66	.55	.72
11	Support colleague	.00	-.01	-.11	.04	.28	.46	.29	.24	.32	.44	–	.57	.45	.41
12	Support supervisor	.01	.03	-.20	.02	.36	.29	.47	.23	.35	.55	.42	–	.62	.56
13	Departmental resources	.17	.02	.01	.04	.35	.29	.36	.55	.42	.57	.42	.51	–	.54
14	Work engagement	.11	.11	-.06	.05	.40	.22	.36	.40	.68	.61	.43	.49	.61	–

Note: $r \geq (-).17$ are significant at the .05 level; [a]: Gender: 1 = female, 2 = male; Worker position: 1 = blue collar work, 2 = lower level white collar work, 3 = self-employed, 4 = job in care or education (e.g., nurse or teacher), 5 = middle level white collar, professional or "free" profession, 6 = higher level white collar worker, management.

Table 3. Results of descriptive discriminant analysis for job status.

Variables	Standardized canonical discriminant function coefficients	Pooled within-group correlations
Job autonomy	.35	.77*
Departmental resources	.81	.93*
Social support colleagues	.03	.45
Social support supervisor	−.27	.48
Work engagement	.14	.64*
Groups	*Function at group centroids*	
Stayers	.15	
Promotion makers	.03	
External movers	−.60	

Note: $R^2 = 95.3$; $\chi^2(10) = 52.39$ ($p < .001$); *largest correlations between variable and function.

($\beta = -.07$, $p < .01$). We compared the fit of an adjusted Model 5 (representing reciprocal effects for the stayers, and reversed effects for the promotion makers and external movers) with the reversed and reciprocal causation Models 3 and 4, and found that the chi-square difference test between Models 3, 4, and 5 produced a non-significant value (M_3 versus M_5: $\Delta\chi^2(4) = 9.02$, $p > .05$; M_4 versus M_5: $\Delta\chi^2(8) = 8.86$, $p > .05$). We can therefore conclude that the results are not identical across the groups.

The standardized effects presented in Figure 1 show that only one normal cross-lagged effect of job autonomy was found for the stayers. This finding is in line with the Job Demands-Resources model, and provides some support for Hypothesis 2. In comparison to the stayers, stronger (subsequently, negative and positive) reversed effects of work engagement on job resources across time were observed among the external movers and especially the promotion makers (supporting Hypotheses 3a and 4a). These results give us information about the causal direction of the relations under study, but do not yet tell us which type of cross-lagged changes and differences took place among the job status groups. We will therefore also examine the across-time mean changes of the different groups.

According to Hypotheses 3b and 4b, we expected that the across-time mean changes of promotion makers would be in line with the positive gain spiral, and the mean changes reported by the external movers would be in line with the refuge hypothesis (e.g., a higher overall level of job resources and work engagement for both groups at Time 2). To examine these hypotheses, a 3 (Job Status: stayers, promotion makers, and external movers) x 2 (Time: Time 1 versus Time 2) repeated measures MANOVA with Time as a within-participants factor and Group as a between-participants factor was carried out. Main effects of Group were found on job autonomy, $F(2, 1025) = 17.73$; social support of supervisors, $F(2, 1025) = 6.68$; departmental resources, $F(2, 1025) = 15.71$; and work engagement, $F(2, 1025) = 8.33$ (all $ps < .05$). Post-hoc least square difference tests revealed that the external movers reported significantly lower scores on work engagement and all job resources (except for colleague support) compared to the stayers and promotion makers.

Table 5 also shows significant Group × Time effects for all variables, revealing that the groups differed significantly in their across-time mean changes. Figures 2–3 present the Times 1–2 means across the groups. Figures 2 and 3 show, in line with Hypotheses 3b and 4b, that the job change groups were successful in positively changing their job autonomy and departmental resources as well as work engagement across time. No significant effects were

Table 4. Fit indices, multi-group structural equation analyses.

Model	Stayers (N=603)	Promotion makers (N=123)	External movers (N=145)	$X^2(df)$	RMSEA	SRMR	GFI	$X^2\Delta(df)$	$X^2\Delta(df)$ M4 versus other models	$X^2\Delta(df)$ M2 versus other models
1	Stability	Stability	Stability	265.77 (155)	.047	.11	.92			
2	Normal	Normal	Normal	246.37 (143)	.047	.11	.92	19.40 (12)		
3	Reversed	Reversed	Reversed	239.37 (143)	.045	.11	.93	26.40** (12)	24.88 (12)*	
4	Reciprocal	Reciprocal	Reciprocal	221.49 (131)	.046	.11	.93	44.28** (24)	17.88 (12)	
5	Reciprocal	Reversed	Reversed	230.35 (139)	.045	.11	.93	35.42** (16)	8.86 (8)	9.02 (4)

Note: $*p < .05$; $**p < .01$.

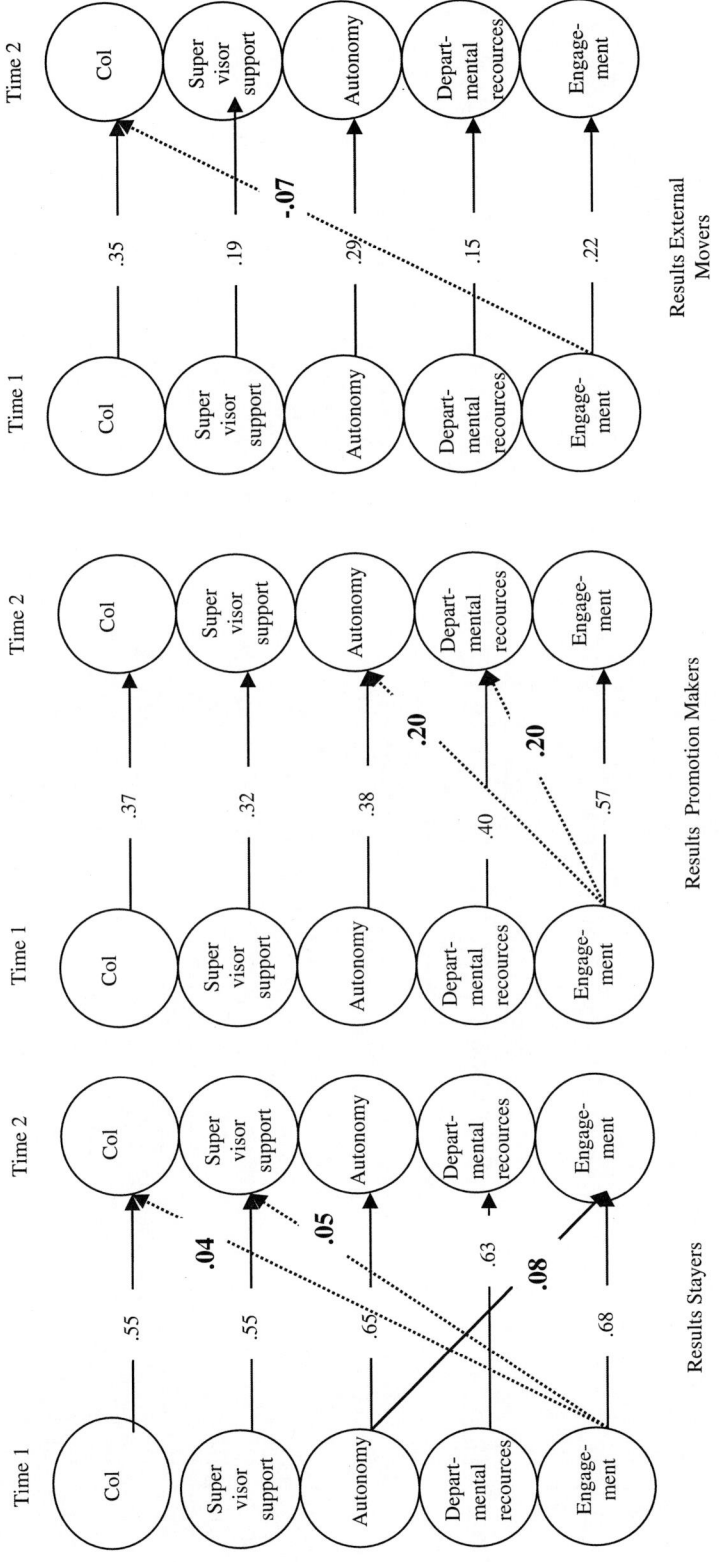

Figure 1. Standardized cross-lagged effects among stayers, promotion makers and external movers.
Note: Results were controlled for influence of covariates age, gender, worker position, and job tenure; Col = social support colleagues, solid arrows refer to normal cross-lagged effects; dotted arrows refer to reversed causal effects.

Table 5. Means and standard deviations (in brackets) of the variables as a function of Time and Group.

Variables	Group 1: Stayers		Group 2: Promotion makers		Group 3: External movers		MANOVA F-values		
	T1	T2	T1	T2	T1	T2	Time	Group	Time × Group
Job autonomy	5.26 (1.29)	5.15[a] (1.32)	5.19 (1.32)	5.51 [a] (1.17)	4.48 (1.57)	4.84 [a] (1.55)	$F_{(1, 1025)}$ =14.22**	$F_{(2, 1025)}$ =17.73**	$F_{(2, 1025)}$ =14.11**
Social support of colleagues	3.14 (.57)	2.99 [a] (.56)	3.10 (.51)	3.03 (.50)	2.95 (.59)	2.99 (.61)	$F_{(1, 1025)}$ =6.28*	$F_{(2, 1025)}$ =2.82, n.s.	$F_{(2, 1025)}$ =8.64**
Social support of Supervisors	2.96 (.74)	2.84 [a] (.73)	3.00 (.75)	3.03 (.64)	2.68 (.82)	2.83 (.79)	$F_{(1, 1025)}$ =.42, n.s.	$F_{(2, 1025)}$ =6.68**	$F_{(2, 1025)}$ =10.08**
Departmental resources	4.66 (1.27)	4.51 [a] (1.33)	4.41 (1.33)	4.68[a] (1.27)	3.73 (1.45)	4.33[a] (1.39)	$F_{(1, 1025)}$ =23.64**	$F_{(2, 1025)}$ =15.71**	$F_{(2, 1025)}$ =28.76**
Work engagement	5.20 (1.21)	5.19 (1.28)	5.15 (1.31)	5.56 [a] (1.09)	4.58 (1.47)	5.15 [a] (1.32)	$F_{(1, 1025)}$ =50.72**	$F_{(2, 1025)}$ =8.33**	$F_{(2, 1025)}$ =22.40**

Note: F-values after controlling for age, gender, worker position, and job tenure; [a] = significant difference between T1 and T2 scores for particular subgroup $p < .01$; n.s. = not significant; Mulitivariate F-test for Time × Group effect was significant ($F_{(10, 2044)} = 7.28$**)
*$p < .05$; **$p < .01$.

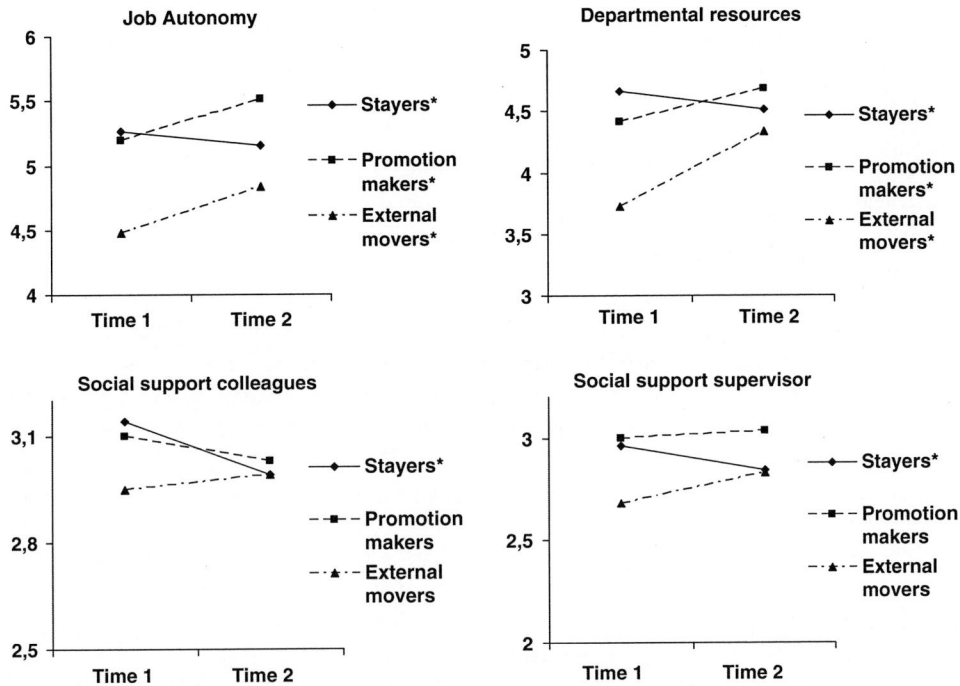

Figure 2.   Times 1 and 2 job resource scores for the stayers, promotion makers, and external movers.

found for colleague and supervisor support. Furthermore, the stayers showed a significant *decrease* in all job resources and a stable work engagement score across time. In sum, these results confirm Hypothesis 3b, as the promotion makers showed significant positive changes after their promotion in terms of job resources and work engagement. We also found support for Hypothesis 4b, as the external movers showed results in line with the "Refuge hypothesis"; starting with the lowest work engagement and job resources, but showing significant positive changes in their job resources as well as work engagement after the job change.

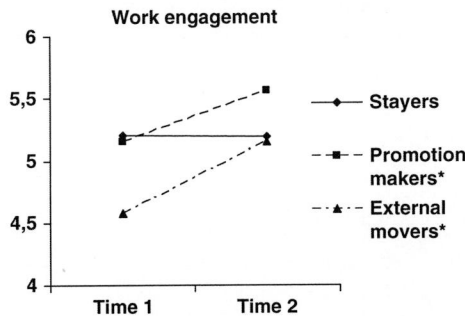

Figure 3.   Times 1 and 2 work engagement scores for the stayers, promotion makers, and external movers.

Discussion

In this paper we focused on three groups: stayers, promotion makers, and external job movers. Longitudinal studies focusing on cross-lagged relations between job resources and work engagement for these three groups are very scarce. We therefore examined these issues in a two-wave (16 month lag) complete panel study among 871 Belgian employees. We started by examining whether the baseline levels of work engagement and job resources were predictive of job status, and found that low departmental resources, low job autonomy, and low work engagement were especially predictive for changing to another company versus staying or making promotions (supporting Hypothesis 1a, and partially supporting Hypothesis 1b). As a consequence, we were able to provide the first longitudinal test and evidence for a relation between low work engagement, job resources, and actual turnover. This finding is consistent with earlier notions that job characteristics as well as psychological states are important predictors in relation to personnel turnover (Griffeth et al., 2000; Schaufeli & Bakker, 2004; Schaufeli et al., 2001).

Subsequently, we tested for differences among the job status groups in their cross-lagged relations between job resources and work engagement. In line with our hypotheses, we found different causal effects for the stayers compared to the external movers. More specifically, among the stayers a normal cross-lagged effect of job autonomy in predicting work engagement across time was found, but also small reversed effects of work engagement in predicting social support of supervisors and colleagues (partially supporting Hypothesis 2; see also Hakanen et al., 2008). The results of the stayers are in line with the assumptions of the Job Demands-Resources model, but also with the reciprocal results found in the studies of Llorens et al. (2007) and Hakanen et al. (2008). In contrast to earlier research, we did not find significant cross-lagged effects of team-related resources or departmental resources for our group of stayers. This finding aligns with models such as Hackman and Oldham's (1980) job characteristics model, in which especially task characteristics like job autonomy are hypothesized to intrinsically stimulate growth and motivation.

Regarding the job change groups or movers, our results revealed different types of significant reversed effects of work engagement on job resources across time for the promotion makers and the external movers (in line with Hypotheses 3a and 4a). More specifically, the expected positive reversed effects of work engagement on job autonomy and departmental resources were found for the promotion makers (in line with Hypothesis 3a), whereas only the expected negative reversed effect for colleague support was observed among the external movers (some support for Hypothesis 4a). These results demonstrate that it is important to disentangle stayers from workers who change jobs, as the aetiology of the observed effects clearly differs. Moreover, the uni-directional view of models like the JD-R model (Bakker & Demerouti, 2007) seems to apply relatively better to stayers compared to job changers.

Besides the direction of the causal effects, we also wanted to examine the reported across-time mean changes in detail. The findings showed that the relatively less engaged as well as the highly engaged workers were able to create a significantly more resourceful work environment after their job change (in line with Hypotheses 3b and 4b). In line with the positive gain spiral hypothesis (cf. Ganster & Schabroeck, 1991), the promotion makers showed the best situation compared to the stayers as well as the external movers, and were able to further improve their job autonomy and departmental resources as well as work engagement across time. In line with the refuge hypothesis (De Lange et al., 2005; Garst et al., 2000), the relatively less engaged external movers were able to significantly increase their job autonomy, departmental resources as well as work engagement after their job change. The only unexpected result was that the stayers reported negative changes in their job resources across time. Van der Velde and Feij (1995) found similar effects in their study when comparing stayers versus job changers, and indicated that these results may reflect a devaluation of the same work situation across time. However, as the stayers are not working in a controlled setting, they may also have experienced real changes that we were not able to exclude or control for in our study.

Combining the effects found for Hypotheses 1–4, we may conclude that the relations among job resources and work engagement are more complex than portrayed in the majority of earlier cross-sectional research. In line with the conservation of resources model (Hobfoll, 2001), our results have shown that workers with strong resource pools (promotion makers) will seek opportunities to further increase their resources. However, in contrast to the "loss spiral" (Hobfoll, 2001) or "drift hypothesis" (Zapf et al., 1996), workers with less strong resource pools can also successfully strive to obtain more resources (as demonstrated by the external movers in this study). It is therefore important to incorporate these positive effects of individual worker behaviour in models like the JD-R model (Bakker & Demerouti, 2007).

Study limitations

At least three limitations of our study deserve some attention. A first limitation is the time lag of 16 months. One could discuss the appropriateness of this time lag. Earlier research (Boswell, Boudreau, & Tichy, 2005; Van der Velde & Feij, 1995) has shown that workers who voluntarily change jobs report an increase in job satisfaction immediately after the job change (the honeymoon effect), followed by a decline in satisfaction after a longer time lag (the hangover effect). With the time lag used, we may have only uncovered the honeymoon period, and may not have captured the full temporal effects of the job change, or potential reversed effects of work engagement, as well as the normal effects of job resources in the new work environment. Fields, Dingman, Roman, and Blum (2005) argue that some of the positive effects reported by the job changers may also reflect *post hoc* justification of the job change (or a so-called cognitive dissonance effect; Festinger, 1957). However, they also argue that variables that predict the likelihood of an employee to make a specific job change (e.g., low work engagement in this study) also reflect the gains that the employee aims to achieve by the job change. This suggests that positive effects probably also reflect substantive changes, rather than just perceptual post hoc justifications.

Another limitation of our study is that we can not fully exclude the explanation that our reported across-time changes of the different groups reflect perceptual changes. For example, due to an increased dedication (and related feelings of enthusiasm), the same job control may be perceived as more useful across time (cf. De Lange et al., 2005). Furthermore, we examined the survivors across time and not the drop-outs. It is important to further examine the drop-outs as these may include the less successful individuals for whom the negative loss spiral or drift-hypothesis might be more valid. In other words, to present a more representative picture, we should also examine the less successful individuals (like the unemployed or those who move to jobs with fewer resources). Nonetheless, we think that the impact of this issue is rather limited, as we did not observe noteworthy differences between the respondents who participated in wave 2 and those who dropped out after wave 1. However, this lack of difference could be due to the specific nature of our respondents: mainly young highly skilled professionals at the beginning of their career. This suggests that it is relevant to replicate our findings among a more representative sample of workers in the future.

Research agenda

From this study, we may derive two main recommendations for future (longitudinal) research examining work engagement:

1. *Investigate different causal relationships among stayers versus movers.* Our study provides evidence for different causal effects among stayers versus movers. We recommend that future research not only examines normal, but also reversed and reciprocal causal relationships between (the same and other) job characteristics (such as job demands, personal job resources) and work engagement. Such research may reveal to which extent the present results generalize to other settings (Rothman & Greenland, 1998).

2. *Test in more detail reversed effects of work engagement.* As this study was one of the first to examine different kinds of reversed effects of work engagement, it is important to validate our results in new more elaborate research. For example, more detailed knowledge about the type of job change should be collected (was it self-determined or imposed, for positive or negative reasons), and other types of job crafters may be selected (such as internal job changers who report self-directed changes). An additional issue relates to workers who are less engaged. Our results suggest that these workers were able to find more resourceful jobs in the future (refuge hypothesis), whereas they could also get involved in a negative gain spiral later on in their career. Future research could try to identify the determinants of both (opposing) processes.

Practical relevance

As this is the first longitudinal study to link (low) work engagement and (limited) job resources to actual personnel turnover, our results confirm the relevance of these variables for organizations in retaining their personnel (Bakker, 2008; Halbesleben & Wheeler, 2008). Employers should be aware that to retain and further motivate one's personnel, it is not only important to provide a positive and resourceful work environment (especially in terms of job autonomy and departmental resources), but also to recognize and understand differences in individual worker behaviour or job crafting processes (Wrzesniewski & Dutton, 2001).

Moreover, it is important to understand how workers perceive the current work environment (in terms of resources, etc.), and whether they need to select new situations to increase their capacities for emotion regulation (Gross, 1998). For highly engaged promotion makers these job crafting processes will very likely result in positive outcomes. However, when workers have become less engaged, the question will arise of whether they should stay or go. Our results suggest that their most likely choice will be to go.

Acknowledgements

We would like to thank Ferdi J. de Goede for his help in conducting the review presented in this study.

References

Note: The references marked with an asterisk were included in the literature review.

Bakker, A.B. (2008). Building engagement in the workplace. In C. Cooper & R. Burke (Eds.), *The peak performing organization*. London: Routledge.

Bakker, A.B. & Demerouti, E. (2007). The Job Demands-Resources model: State of the art. *Journal of Managerial Psychology, 22*, 309–328.

*Bakker, A.B., Demerouti, E. & Schaufeli, W.B. (2005). The crossover of burnout and work engagement among working couples. *Human Relations, 58*, 661–689.

*Bakker, A.B., Hakanen, J.J., Demerouti, E. & Xanthopoulou, D. (2007). Job resources boost work engagement, particularly when job demands are high. *Journal of Educational Psychology, 99*, 274–284.

Bakker, A.B., Schaufeli, W.B., Leiter, M.P., & Taris, T.W. (2008). Work engagement: An emerging concept in occupational health psychology. *Work & Stress, 22*, 187–200.

*Bakker, A.B., Van Emmerik, H., & Eeuwema, M.C. (2006). Crossover of burnout and engagement in work teams. *Work and Occupations, 33*, 464–489.

Bentler, P.M. & Chou, C.P. (1987). Practical issues in structural modeling. *Sociological Methods and Research, 16*, 78–117.

Boswell, W.R., Boudreau, J.W. & Tichy, J. (2005). The relationship between employee job change and job satisfaction: The honeymoon-hangover effect. *Journal of Applied Psychology, 90*, 882–892.

Byrne, B.M. (2002). *Structural equation modeling with AMOS*. Mahwah, NJ: Lawrence Erlbaum.

Cooper, C.L. (2005). Guest editorial: Stress and health: A positive direction. *Stress and Health, 21*, 73–75.

De Cuyper, N., Notelaers, G., & De Witte, H. (in press). Transitioning between temporary and permanent employment: A two-wave study on the entrapment, the stepping stone and the selection hypothesis. *Journal of Occupational and Organizational Psychology*.

De Lange, A.H., Taris, T.W., Kompier, M.A.J., Houtman, I.L.D. & Bongers, P.M. (2004). Work characteristics and psychological well-being. Testing normal, reversed and reciprocal relationships within the 4-wave SMASH study. *Work & Stress, 18*, 149–166.

De Lange, A.H., Taris, T.W., Kompier, M.A.J., Houtman, I.L.D. & Bongers, P.M. (2005). Different mechanisms to explain the reversed effects of mental health on work characteristics. *Scandinavian Journal of Work, Environment and Health, 31*, 3–14.

Deci, W.L. & Ryan, R.M. (1985). *Intrinsic motivation and self-determination in human behavior*. New York: Plenum.

Demerouti, E., Bakker, A.B., Nachreiner, F. & Schaufeli, W.B. (2001). The job demands-resources model of burnout. *Journal of Applied Psychology, 86*, 499–512.

Dormann, C. & Zapf, D. (2002). Social stressors at work, irritation, and depressive symptoms: Accounting for unmeasured third variables in a multi-wave study. *Journal of Occupational and Organizational Psychology, 75*, 33–58.

Ettner, S.L. & Gryzwacz, J.G. (2001). Workers' perceptions of how jobs affect health: A social ecological perspective. *Journal of Occupational Health Psychology, 6*, 101–113.

Festinger, L. (1957). *A theory of cognitive dissonance*. Standford, CA: Standford University Press.

Fields, D., Dingman, M.E., Roman, P.M. & Blum, T.C. (2005). Exploring predictors of alternative job changes. *Journal of Occupational and Organizational Psychology, 78*, 63–82.

Fredrickson, B.L. (2001). The role of positive emotions in positive psychology: The Broaden-and-Built theory of positive emotions. *American Psychologist, 56*, 218–226.

Frese, M. (1985). Stress at work and psychosomatic complaints: A causal interpretation. *Journal of Applied Psychology, 70*, 314–328.

Frese, M., Garst, H. & Fay, D. (2007). Making things happen: reciprocal relationships between work characteristics and personal initiative in a four-wave longitudinal structural equation model. *Journal of Applied Psychology, 92*, 1084–1102.

Gable, S.L. & Haidt, J. (2005). What (and why) is positive psychology. *Review of General Psychology, 9,* 103–110.

Ganster, D.C. & Schabroeck, J. (1991). Work stress and employee health. *Journal of Management, 17,* 235–271.

Garst, H., Frese, M. & Molenaar, P.C.M. (2000). The temporal factor of change in stressor-strain relationships: A growth curve model on a longitudinal study in East Germany. *Journal of Applied Psychology, 85,* 417–438.

González-Romá, V., Schaufeli, W.B., Bakker, A. & Lloret, S. (2006). Burnout and engagement: Independent factors or opposite poles? *Journal of Vocational Behavior, 68,* 165–174.

Griffeth, R.W., Hom, P.W. & Gaertner, B. (2000). A meta-analysis of antecedents and correlates of employee turnover: update, moderator tests and research implications for the next millennium. *Journal of Management, 26,* 463–488.

Gross, J.J. (1998). The emerging field of emotion regulation: an integrative review. *Review of General Psychology, 2,* 271–299.

Hackman, J.R. & Oldham, G.R. (1980). *Work redesign.* Reading, MA: Addison-Wesley.

*Hakanen, J.J., Bakker, A.B., & Schaufeli, W.B. (2006). Burnout and work engagement among teachers. *Journal of School Psychology, 43,* 495–513.

Hakanen, J.J., Schaufeli, W.B., & Ahola, K. (2008). The Job Demands-Resources model: A three-year cross-lagged study of burnout, depression, commitment, and work engagement. *Work & Stress, 22,* 224–241.

Halbesleben, J.R.B. (2006). Sources of social support and burnout: A meta-analytic test of the conservation of resources model. *Journal of Applied Psychology, 91,* 1134–1145.

Halbesleben, J.R.B., & Wheeler, A.R. (2008). The relative roles of engagement and embeddedness in predicting job performance and intention to leave. *Work & Stress, 22,* 242–256.

*Hallberg, U.E., & Schaufeli, W.B. (2006). "Same same" but different? Can work engagement be discriminated from job involvement and organizational commitment? *European Psychologist, 11,* 119–127.

*Hallberg, U.E., Johansson, G., & Schaufeli, W.B. (2007). Type A behaviour and work situation: Associations with burnout and work engagement. *Scandinavian Journal of Psychology, 48,* 135–142.

Hobfoll, S.E. (1985). The limitations of social support in the stress process. In I.G. Sarason & B.R. Sarason (Eds.), *Social support: Theory, research and applications* (pp. 391–414). Boston: Martinus Nijhoff.

Hobfoll, S.E. (2001). The influence of culture, community, and the nested-self in the stress process: Advancing conservation resources theory. *Applied Psychology: An International Review, 50,* 337–370.

*Jackson, L.T.B., Rothmannm S., & Van de Vijver, F.J.R. (2006). A model of work-related well-being for educators in South Africa. *Stress & Health, 22,* 263–274.

James, L.R., Mulaik, S.A. & Brett, J.M. (1982). *Causal analysis: Assumptions, models and data.* Beverly Hills, CA: Sage.

Jöreskog, K.G. & Sörbom, D. (1993). *Lisrel-8 (user's manual).* Chicago: Scientific Software.

Kasl, S.V. & Jones, B.A. (2003). An epidemiological perspective on research design, measurement and surveillance strategies. In J.C. Quick & L.E. Tetrick (Eds.), *Handbook of occupational health psychology* (pp. 379–398). Washington: American Psychological Association.

Kelloway, K.E. (1998). *Using Lisrel for structural equation modeling: A researcher's guide.* London: Sage Publications.

*Llorens, S., Bakker, A.B., Schaufeli, W.B., & Salanova, M. (2006). Testing the robustness of the Job Demands-Resources Model. *International Journal of Stress Management, 13,* 378–391.

*Llorens, S., Schaufeli, W., Bakker, A. & Salanova, M. (2007). Does a positive gain spiral of resources, efficacy beliefs and engagement exist? *Computers in Human Behavior, 23,* 825–841.

Marmot, M.G. & Madge, N. (1987). An epidemiological perspective on stress and health. In S.V. Kasl & C.L. Cooper (Eds.), *Research methods in stress and health psychology* (pp. 3–26). New York: John Wiley & Sons Ltd.

Martin, A.J. (2005). The role of positive psychology in enhancing satisfaction, motivation and productivity in the workplace. *Journal of Organizational Behavior Management, 24,* 113–132.

Mauno, S., Kinnunen, U., Mäkikangas, A. & Nätti, J. (2005). Psychological consequences of fixed-term employment and perceived job insecurity among health care staff. *European Journal of Work and Organizational Psychology, 14,* 209–238.

*Mauno, S., Kinnunen, U. & Ruokolainen, M. (2007). Job demands and resources as antecedents of work engagement: A longitudinal study. *Journal of Vocational Behaviour, 70,* 149–171.

*Montgomery, A.J., Peeters, M.C.W., Schaufeli, W.B., & Den Ouden, M. (2003). Work–home interference among newspaper managers: its relationship with burnout and engagement. *Anxiety, Stress, and Coping, 16,* 195–211.

Ployhart, R.E. (2006). Staffing in the 21st century: New challenges and strategic opportunities. *Journal of Management, 32,* 868–879.

*Richardson, A.M., Burke, R.J., & Martinussen, M. (2006). Work and health outcomes among police officers: The mediating role of police cynicism and engagement. *International Journal of Stress Management, 13,* 555–574.

Rothman, K.J. & Greenland, S. (1998). *Modern epidemiology.* Philadelphia: Lippincott-Raven Publishers.

Ryan, R.M. & Frederick, C.M. (1997). On energy, personality, and health: Subjective vitality as dynamic reflection of well-being. *Journal of Personality, 65,* 529–565.

*Salanova, M., Agut, S. & Peiró, J.M. (2005). Linking organizational resources and work engagement to employee performance and customer loyalty: The mediation of service climate. *Journal of Applied Psychology, 90,* 1217–1227.

Salanova, M., Bakker, A.B. & Llorens, S. (2006). Flow at work: evidence for an upward spiral of personal and organizational resources. *Journal of Happiness Studies, 7,* 1–22.

*Schaufeli, W.B. & Bakker, A.B. (2004). Job demands, job resources, and their relationship with burnout and engagement: A multi-sample study. *Journal of Organizational Behavior, 25,* 293–315.

Schaufeli, W.B., & Bakker, A.B. (2008). The conceptualization and measurement of work engagement: A review. In A.B. Bakker & M.P. Leiter (Eds.), *Work engagement: Recent developments in theory and research.* New York: Psychology Press.

Schaufeli, W.B., & Bakker, A.B. (in press). *The Utrecht work engagement scale. Preliminary manual.* Utrecht University.

Schaufeli, W.B., Salanova, M., González-Romá, V. & Bakker, A.B. (2002). The measurement of engagement and burnout: A two sample confirmatory factor analytic approach. *Journal of Happiness Studies, 3,* 71–92.

Schaufeli, W.B., Taris, T.W., Le Blanc, P., Peeters, M., Bakker, A.B. & De Jonge, J. (2001). Maakt arbeid gezond? Op zoek naar de bevlogen werknemer [Does work make happy? In search of the engaged worker]. *De Psycholoog, 36,* 422–428.

Schumacker, R.E. & Lomax, R.G. (1996). *A beginner's guide to structural equation modeling.* Mahwah, NJ: Lawrence Erlbaum.

*Sonnentag, S. (2003). Recovery, work engagement, and proactive behaviour: A new look at the interface between nonwork and work. *Journal of Applied Psychology, 88,* 518–528.

Stevens, J. (1996). *Applied multivariate statistics for the social sciences.* Mahwah, NJ: Lawrence Erlbaum.

Taris, T.W., Bok, I.A. & Caljé, D.G. (1998). On the relation between job characteristics and depression: A longitudinal study. *International Journal of Stress Management, 5,* 157–167.

Van den Broeck, A., Vansteenkiste, M., De Witte, H., & Lens, W., (2008). Explaining the relationships between job characteristics, burnout, and engagement: The role of basic psychological need satisfaction. *Work & Stress, 22,* 277–294.

Vander Elst, T., Eertmans, A., Taeymans, S., & De Witte, H. (2008). *The short-inventory on stress and well-being: a psychometric evaluation.* Manuscript submitted for publication.

Velde, van der, M.E.G., & Feij, J.A. (1995). Change of work perceptions and work outcomes as a result of voluntary and involuntary job change. *Journal of Organizational and Occupational Psychology, 68,* 273–290.

Veldhoven, van, M., & Meijman, T. (1994). *Het meten van psychosociale arbeidsbelasting met een vragenlijst: de vragenlijst beleving en beoordeling van de arbeid (VBBA)* [The measurement of psychosocial job demands with a questionnaire: The questionnaire on the experience and evaluation of work]. Amsterdam: Nederlands Instituut voor Arbeidsomstandigheden.

Warr, P. (2007). *Work, happiness, and unhappiness.* London: Lawrence Erlbaum Associates.

Wrzesniewski, A. & Dutton, J.E. (2001). Crafting a job: revisioning employees as active crafters of their work. *Academy of Management Review, 26,* 179–201.

*Xanthopoulou, D., Bakker, A.B., Demerouti, E. & Schaufeli, W.B. (2007). The role of personal resources in the job demands-resources model. *International Journal of Stress Management, 14,* 121–141.

Zapf, D., Dormann, C. & Frese, M. (1996). Longitudinal studies in organizational stress research: A review of the literature with reference to methodological issues. *Journal of Occupational Health Psychology, 1,* 145–169.

Are job and personal resources associated with work ability 10 years later? The mediating role of work engagement

Auli Airila[a], Jari J. Hakanen[a], Wilmar B. Schaufeli[b], Ritva Luukkonen[c], Anne Punakallio[d] and Sirpa Lusa[d]

[a]Development of Work and Organizations, Finnish Institute of Occupational Health, Helsinki, Finland; [b]Department of Social and Organizational Psychology, University of Utrecht, Utrecht, The Netherlands; [c]Creating Solutions, Finnish Institute of Occupational Health, Helsinki, Finland; [d]Health and Work Ability, Finnish Institute of Occupational Health, Helsinki, Finland

Using a two-wave 10-year longitudinal design, this study examined the motivational process proposed by the Job Demands-Resources (JD-R) model. The aim was to examine whether work engagement acts as a mediator between job resources (i.e. supervisory relations, interpersonal relations and task resources) and personal resources (self-esteem) on the one hand and future work ability (i.e. a worker's functional ability to do their job) on the other. The second aim was to investigate the mediating role of engagement between past work ability and future work ability. Structural equation modelling was used to test the mediation hypotheses among Finnish firefighters ($N = 403$). As hypothesized, engagement at T2 fully mediated the impact of job and personal resources at T1 on work ability at T2. In addition, the effect of work ability at T1 on work ability at T2 was partially mediated by engagement at T2. These results indicate that job and personal resources may have long-term effects on engagement, and consequently on work ability, thus expanding on the propositions of the JD-R model. The results show a dual role of work ability, as a health-related resource that may foster engagement and an outcome driven by the motivational process proposed by the JD-R model.

Introduction

The well-established Job Demands-Resources (JD-R) model (Demerouti, Bakker, Nachreiner, & Schaufeli, 2001) assumes that work characteristics, such as job demands and job resources, have either positive or negative effects on employee well-being. The basic assumption of the JD-R model is that two distinct psychological processes — the health-impairment process and the motivational process — are differently related to well-being. Firstly, the health-impairment process assumes that job demands lead to burnout, and consequently to ill-health. Secondly, the motivational process assumes that job resources lead to work engagement, which, in turn, has a positive effect on organizational outcomes. According to the later formulations of the JD-R model, personal resources, such as self-esteem, may have similar motivational potential to that of job resources (Xanthopoulou, Bakker, Demerouti, & Schaufeli, 2007). However, one limitation of the JD-R model has been its neglect to elucidate the relationship between job and personal resources and health-related outcomes. Nevertheless, the motivational process initiated by job and personal resources, through engagement, may also lead to positive health-related outcomes (e.g. Hakanen & Roodt, 2010), such as work ability.

Work ability refers to workers' ability to carry out their work, that is, having the occupational competence, the health required for the job and the occupational virtues that are required for managing the work tasks (Tengland, 2011). Thus, work ability refers to functional capacity to meet the requirements of the job. So far, work ability research has not studied the motivational aspects of human resources with the same intensity as it has biographical and life-style factors (e.g. age, alcohol consumption, physical exercise, BMI) and work-related factors (e.g. mental and physical work demands, management) (for a review, see Van den Berg, Elders, Zwart, & Burdorf, 2009), despite the fact that affective-motivational factors such as work engagement are considered essential factors related to work ability (e.g. Ilmarinen, 2009). To conclude, it is not yet clear what the relationships are between engagement and work ability, and between self-esteem and work ability; and the long-term impacts that both job and personal resources may have on work ability via engagement.

Therefore, in the present study, using the Conservation of Resources (COR) theory (Hobfoll, 1989), the Broaden-and-Build (BaB) theory (Fredrickson, 2001) and self-enhancement theory (Jones, 1973) as theoretical frameworks, we examined the motivational properties of job and personal resources in the JD-R model in a sample of Finnish firefighters. Based on those theories, we argue that both job and personal resources are significantly related to future work engagement, and consequently, to work ability. More specifically, we examined whether work engagement acts as a mediator between job resources and self-esteem (a personal resource) on the one hand, and work ability on the other. In addition, we examined whether work engagement mediates the effect of past work ability on future work ability. Thus, we investigated the dual role of work ability in the motivational process as proposed in the JD-R model. More particularly, we studied the role of work ability as a health-related outcome of the motivational process, and simultaneously its role as a health-related resource that may boost work engagement and consequently predict not only directly but also indirectly future work ability across a 10-year follow-up period.

Job resources and work engagement in the JD-R model

The basic assumption of the JD-R model is that job resources are positively related to work engagement, which, in turn, is related to positive outcomes, thus constituting a motivational process (Bakker & Demerouti, 2007). As such, job resources refer to those physical, psychological, social or organizational aspects of the job that may help to achieve work goals, reduce job demands and the related physiological and psychological costs, and stimulate personal growth and development (Demerouti et al., 2001). Additionally, work engagement refers to an affective-motivational state of work-related well-being that is characterized by vigour, dedication and absorption (Schaufeli, Salanova, González-Roma, & Bakker, 2002).

In the current study among firefighters, we included three job resources that prior studies have identified as important resources for this professional group: (1) *supervisory support* (e.g. Haslam & Mallon, 2003; Mitani, Fujita, Nakata, & Shirakawa, 2006); (2) *supportive interpersonal relations* (e.g. Saijo, Ueno, & Hashimoto, 2007); and (3) *task resources* (e.g. Lusa, Punakallio, Luukkonen, & Louhevaara, 2006). Self-Determination Theory (SDT; Deci & Ryan, 2000; Van den Broeck, Vansteenkiste, de Witte, & Lens, 2008) offers a plausible explanation for the choice of the three selected job resources. According to SDT, intrinsic motivation will flourish if three basic psychological needs — autonomy, competence and relatedness — are satisfied. For firefighters, autonomy may be related to their ability to make decisions concerning their work tasks (i.e. task resources); competence may be related to their opportunities to use their skills at work (i.e. task resources); and social support from colleagues and supervisors to the relatedness need of SDT (i.e. supervisory support and interpersonal relations), all of which are consistently shown to be related to work engagement (e.g. Hakanen & Roodt, 2010; Van den Broeck et al., 2008).

COR theory (Hobfoll, 1989) describes pathways from job resources to employee health. Firstly, the basic tenet of the resource-orientated COR theory is that people strive to retain, protect and build resources that they value. Moreover, these resources, such as conditions (i.e. job resources) or personal characteristics (i.e. self-esteem) are salient in gaining new resources and in enhancing health. More precisely, those with greater resources are less vulnerable to stress, and additionally they are more capable of future resource gain, and consequently will have better protection against ill-health. To summarize, the COR theory, alongside the JD-R model, assumes that high levels of resources can be beneficial for health (and work ability) in the long term.

Empirically, the motivational process of the JD-R model, leading from job resources through engagement to positive organizational outcomes, has been convincingly supported (for an overview, see Schaufeli & Taris, 2014). For example, organizational outcomes such as customer loyalty (Salanova, Agut, & Peiró, 2005), organizational commitment (Hakanen, Schaufeli, & Ahola, 2008) and innovativeness (Hakanen, Perhoniemi, & Toppinen-Tanner, 2008) have been examined. In contrast, the link between job resources via work engagement to *health-related* outcomes, such as work ability, has rarely been investigated. Nevertheless, based on the COR theory we assume that job resources may also be positively related to health-related outcomes via engagement. In fact, some evidence exists on the positive association between job resources and/or engagement and health-related outcomes (e.g. Hakanen & Schaufeli, 2012; Parzefall & Hakanen, 2010). Additional evidence corroborates the positive relations between work engagement and health (e.g. Langelaan, Bakker, Schaufeli, van Rhenen, & van Doornen, 2006; Seppälä et al., 2012) and between work engagement and work ability (e.g. Airila, Hakanen, Punakallio, Lusa, & Luukkonen, 2012; Hakanen, Bakker, & Schaufeli, 2006).

In addition, previous studies have shown a long-term impact of resources on well-being, thus supporting the assumption of COR theory of a slow accumulation process resulting in long-term resource gains. For example, a study among the Finnish working population (Hakanen, Bakker, & Jokisaari, 2011) showed that skill variety (a job resource) negatively predicted burnout 13 years later, even after controlling for the concurrent levels of skill variety. In addition, a study among Dutch employees showed that various job and personal resources were positively related to work engagement over a follow-up period of 18 months (Xanthopoulou, Bakker, Demerouti, & Schaufeli, 2009). Similarly, Hakanen, Peeters, and Perhoniemi (2011) found that various job resources predicted both work engagement and work-family enrichment over a three-year follow-up period, further supporting the notion of long-term resource gain processes. Taken together, these findings suggest that the motivational process proposed by the JD-R model may also lead to better health — although the primary health outcomes may often follow the health-impairment pathway. Therefore, based on theoretical reasoning as well as earlier empirical findings, we formulate the following hypothesis:

Hypothesis 1: Job resources at T1 will be positively related to work ability at T2 through work engagement at T2. In other words, work engagement will mediate the relationship between job resources and future work ability.

Personal resources in the JD-R model

A more recent formulation of the JD-R model proposes that personal resources may have similar motivational potential to that of job resources and may be positively related to work engagement, and consequently to positive work-related outcomes (Xanthopoulou et al., 2007). By definition, personal resources are positive self-evaluations that are linked to resilience, and refer to an individual's sense of ability to successfully control and impact on his or her environment (Hobfoll, Johnson, Ennis, & Jackson, 2003). In the current study, we included self-esteem as a typical personal resource that may be beneficial for achieving positive work-related outcomes (e.g. Hobfoll, 2001). Self-esteem refers to a positive evaluation of one's worth, significance and ability as a person (Janssen, Schaufeli, & Houkes, 1999; Rosenberg, 1965). According to Hobfoll (2001), self-esteem can be viewed as a personal characteristic that is valued in its own right. Indeed, self-esteem — as a personal resource — may play an important role in human functioning in two ways.

First, COR theory (Hobfoll, 1989) proposes that personal resources (e.g. self-esteem) tend to generate other resources, which, in their turn, may result in better well-being. More precisely, according to COR theory, the loss or gain of self-esteem results in stress or well-being, respectively. In a similar vein, Rosenberg, Schooler, Schoenbach, and Rosenberg (1995) have emphasized the value of global self-esteem as a predictor of (psychological) well-being. Secondly, self-enhancement theory (Jones, 1973; see also Rosenberg et al., 1995) provides a theoretical explanation for the underlying mechanism that links self-esteem to health-related outcomes. According to this theory, people strive to protect and enhance their feelings of self-worth (i.e. self-esteem). This maintenance of self-esteem leads to self-protective motives, and thus to the beneficial development of well-being. Therefore, based on these theories we assume that self-esteem — as a personal resource — is an antecedent of work engagement (i.e. work-related well-being), and consequently related to work ability.

Indeed, some evidence exists of the positive relationship between self-esteem and well-being (for a review, see Baumeister, Campbell, Krueger, & Vohs, 2003). For example, in their 10-year longitudinal study of university students, Salmela-Aro and Nurmi (2007) found that self-esteem predicted work engagement, thereby suggesting that resource gain processes can take place over a long time period. Research findings also show that high self-esteem may protect from burnout (Alarcon, Eschleman, & Bowling,

2009; Janssen et al., 1999; Kalimo, Pahkin, Mutanen, & Toppinen-Tanner, 2003). Together these studies suggest that a high level of self-esteem helps employees to cope successfully with stressors at work, and consequently, may lead to better health and well-being. Tellingly, to our knowledge, the link between self-esteem and *work ability* has not yet been examined, despite the fact that COR theory and self-enhancement theory provide a plausible theoretical framework for explaining the relationship between these variables. Thus, based on these three approaches, it can be assumed that employees who see themselves as worthy, significant and able as a person may also be more willing to put effort into their work tasks, and become fully involved in their work. As a result, their work ability will also be better than that of employees with lower levels of self-esteem. Therefore, we formulate the following hypothesis:

Hypothesis 2: Self-esteem at T1 will be positively related to work ability at T2 through work engagement at T2. In other words, work engagement will mediate the relationship between self-esteem and future work ability.

Work ability as a health-related resource in the JD-R model

Traditionally, in the JD-R model health-related indicators are considered to be outcomes of the health-impairment process. However, health-related outcomes may themselves be important resources that boost work engagement and consequently further improve health and well-being. In fact, The World Health Organization (WHO) defines health as a positive concept including physical, mental and social well-being, that is, "a resource for everyday life" rather than the objective of living (WHO, 1986). Thus, health can be conceptualized as a kind of capital in which individuals may invest in order to achieve positive future health outcomes (Williamson & Carr, 2009). In a similar vein, it can be argued that work ability is a health-related resource that is likely to be related to future well-being.

The Broaden-and-Build (BaB) theory of positive emotions (Fredrickson, 2001) provides a possible theoretical explanation for the mechanism that links work engagement and work ability. According to this theory, positive emotions broaden peoples' thought-action repertoires, build their enduring personal resources and consequently lead to better well-being (see also Ouweneel, Le Blanc, Schaufeli, & Van Wijhe, 2012). Thus, based on the build hypotheses of the BaB theory, work engagement can be assumed to build health-related resources, such as work ability. In addition, and in line with COR theory, BaB theory proposes that emotions and well-being affect each other reciprocally (i.e. gain or upward spirals), supporting the assumption of mutually positive relationships between work ability and work engagement.

Empirically, there is convincing evidence supporting the role of work ability as a resource that may have beneficial effects on well-being and other health-related variables also in the long term. For example, Seitsamo et al. (2011) showed that work ability was a strong predictor of later-life health in a 28-year longitudinal study among Finnish municipal workers. Similarly, Ahlstrom, Grimby-Ekman, Hagberg, and Dellve (2010) found that work ability predicted future health among women working in human service organizations. Feldt, Hyvönen, Mäkikangas, Kinnunen, and Kokko (2009) in their turn showed that work ability of Finnish managers was related to job involvement and organizational commitment — both constructs that are closely related to work engagement.

Thus, based on BaB theory and on earlier research findings, we argue that work ability can be viewed as a health-related resource that fosters a high level of positive energy (vigour), strong identification (dedication) and strong focus (absorption) on one's work. Hence, we assume that good work ability is likely to influence work engagement, which, in its turn, may improve future work ability. Thus, we formulate our next hypothesis:

Hypothesis 3: Work ability at T1 will be positively related to work engagement at T2, which in its turn will be positively related to subsequent work ability at T2. In other words, work engagement will partially mediate the impact of work ability at T1 on work ability at T2.

The research model is graphically illustrated in Figure 1.

Method

Procedure and participants

The data is part of a questionnaire study among Finnish firefighters conducted in 1996, 1999 and 2009. In this study, we use the data from 1999 and in 2009 which include the variables of interest in the present study. The 10-year interval between data collections was determined by practical decisions and financial arrangements that the researchers could not influence. This long time interval offered the possibility to study the effect of the slow process of personal resource accumulation. In 1999, 1124 questionnaires were posted, and 72% ($n = 794$) were returned. At follow-up 10 years later, 68% ($n = 721$) returned the questionnaire. The research process is reported in detail elsewhere (Lusa et al., 2006; Lusa, Punakallio, & Luukkonen, 2011).

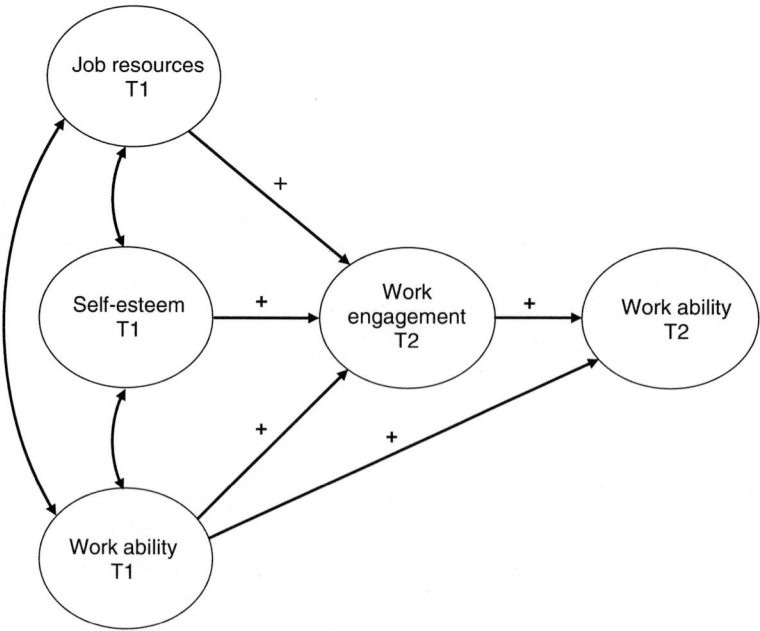

Figure 1. The theoretical model.

The study population of the current research consisted of professional operational firefighters who responded to the questionnaires in both 1999 (T1) and 2009 (T2), and were still employed in their profession (N = 403). All participants were men. At T2, the average age of the study population was 48.5 (range 35–62, SD = 5.4). The large majority (88%, n = 315) had firefighter qualifications, 29% (n = 105) had a sub-officer qualification and 10% (n = 35) had a fire chief qualification. Mean work experience in fire and rescue services was 25.3 years (range 3–39, SD = 5.8). Finally, at T2, 2% (n = 9) were not participating in operative tasks.

Of the respondents from 1999, 148 dropped out and did not participate in the study in 2009. Two-sample t-tests indicated that the dropouts were slightly older (mean age 39.9 vs. 38.5 years), had lower education (primary school education 29% vs. 18%) and had poorer work ability (mean score 7.5 vs. 8.1, score range 0–10) than those who responded at both times. By contrast, two-sample Wilcoxon tests revealed that the dropouts and the participants did *not* significantly differ in relation to self-esteem (mean value 34.85 vs. 34.31; score range 10–40), supervisory relations (mean value 3.78 vs. 3.73), interpersonal relations (mean value 3.95 vs. 3.97) or task resources (mean value 3.19 vs. 3.05; all three ranges 1–5).

Measurements

Job resources. The three job resources at T1 — supervisory relations, interpersonal relations and task resources — were adapted from the Occupational Stress Questionnaire, which is well validated in Finland (Elo, Leppänen, Lindström, & Ropponen, 1992). *Supervisory relations* included five items covering supervisory support, supervisory control and relationships between employees and supervisors. An example item is "Do you get support and help from your supervisor when needed?". *Interpersonal relations* consisted of four items: conflicts between employees, conflicts between younger and older workers, cooperation in one's work-unit and relationships between employees. An example item is "Do conflicts between employees affect your work?". *Task resources* included three items: decision making on issues concerning one's tasks, opportunities to use one's knowledge and skills at work and feedback on success in work tasks. An example item is "Can you use your knowledge and skills at work?". All job resource items were rated on a five-point scale ranging from 1 (*not at all/practically never*) to 5 (*very much*). A high score indicates a perception of supportive and co-operative supervision, positive interaction and co-operation between co-workers, task autonomy, opportunities for skill utilization and feedback.

Self-esteem. Self-esteem at T1 was measured using the Rosenberg Self-Esteem Scale (Rosenberg, 1965) consisting of 10 items. Rosenberg's self-report scale is one of the most widely used measures of self-esteem (Marsh, 1996). It includes both positive (e.g. "On the whole, I am satisfied with myself") and negative (e.g. "At times I think I am no good at all") items. All items were rated on a four-point scale ranging from 1 (*strongly disagree*) to 4 (*strongly agree*).

Work engagement. Work engagement at T2 was measured by the short version of the Utrecht Work Engagement Scale, UWES (Schaufeli, Bakker, & Salanova, 2006), consisting of nine items, with three sub-scales: vigour (e.g. "At my work, I feel bursting with energy"), dedication (e.g. "My job inspires me") and absorption (e.g. "I am immersed in my work"). Each of the dimensions was assessed using three items. The items were rated on a seven-point frequency-based scale ranging from 0 (*never*) to 6 (*daily*).

Work ability. Work ability at T1 and T2 was measured by one question with a scale from 0 to 10: "Assume that your work ability at its best has had a value of 10. How many points would you give your current work ability? (0 means that currently you cannot work at all)". This single-item question was derived from the Work Ability Index (WAI) questionnaire (Tuomi, Ilmarinen, Jahkola, Katajarinne, & Tulkki, 1998), a valid measure of work ability (van den Berg et al., 2009). Prior studies have indicated a strong association between the total WAI-score and the single-item indicator (e.g. Ahlstrom et al., 2010). In addition, both the total WAI and the single-item question have shown similar patterns of associations with diverse health-related outcomes (e.g. Ahlstrom et al., 2010). Thus, a single-item question of work ability is a good alternative to the rather complex measure of total WAI-index, and has been widely used in Finnish work life and health surveys (e.g. Kauppinen et al., 2010).

Score ranges for all variables are given in Table 1.

Data analysis

To test our hypotheses, we used structural equation modelling (SEM) techniques with maximum likelihood (ML) estimation and the AMOS 18.0 software package (Arbuckle, 2009). After testing the measurement model, we tested five different structural equation models. These were, firstly, the *hypothesized mediation model* (M1) in which work engagement fully mediates the relationships between job resources and self-esteem at T1 and work ability at T2, and partially mediates the relationship between work ability at T1 and work ability at T2; secondly, the *partial mediation model* (M2) which includes both the indirect (via engagement) and direct relationships between job resources and self-esteem at T1 and work ability at T2; thirdly, the *direct model* (M3) in which both job resources and self-esteem at T1 relate to work ability at T2 without the mediating role of work engagement, and work engagement relates to work ability at T2. In the fourth model, the *alternative direct model* (M4), job resources, self-esteem and work ability at T1 simultaneously relate to work engagement at T2 and work ability at T2. Thus, M4 includes three variables from T1 and two parallel outcomes at T2, and no mediators. Fifthly and finally, we tested *the alternative model* (M5) in which work ability at T1 is not related to work engagement, whereas the relationships between job resources and self-esteem at T1, and work ability at T2 are fully mediated by work engagement. Thus, this model was similar to the M1 except for removing the link between work ability at T1 and work engagement at T2.

The latent job resources variable was indicated by supervisory relations, interpersonal relations and task resources. After conducting an exploratory factor analysis, two scales

Table 1. Means, standard deviations and correlations between the study variables ($N = 403$).

Variables	Range	M	SD	1	2	3	4	5	6	7	8
1. Self-rated work ability T1	0–10	8.06	1.23	–							
2. Supervisory relations T1	1–5	3.78	.78	.15*	(.80)						
3. Interpersonal relations T1	1–5	3.95	.77	.10*	.49**	(.72)					
4. Task resources T1	1–5	3.19	.66	.08	.48**	.18**	(.68)				
5. Self-esteem T1	10–40	34.85	3.98	.19**	.23**	.16***	.26**	(.81)			
6. Vigour T2	0–6	3.90	1.48	.19**	.24**	.19***	.27***	.21**	(.89)		
7. Dedication T2	0–6	3.98	1.51	.17**	.18**	.17***	.26**	.23**	.90**	(.90)	
8. Absorption T2	0–6	3.30	1.58	.08	.16**	.16***	.23**	.12*	.78**	.81**	(.90)
9. Self-rated work ability T2	0–10	7.13	1.71	.33**	.18**	.05	.12*	.20**	.33**	.31**	.25**

Note: Cronbach's alphas are on the diagonal in parentheses.
*$p < .05$; **$p < .01$.

based on positive and negative items measuring self-esteem emerged, and they were used as indicators of the latent self-esteem factor. Work engagement was indicated by vigour, dedication and absorption scales. Work ability was based on a single-item indicator.

Model fit was evaluated using goodness-of-fit indices and conventional rules of thumb for their cut-offs. To test our hypotheses, we used the Chi-square (χ^2) test for goodness-of-fit, and compared the means of the chi-square difference test of different models. In addition, we examined the Root Mean Square Error of Approximation (RMSEA), the Comparative Fit Index (CFI) and the Tucker-Lewis Index (TLI). For RMSEA, values below .05 are indicative of a good fit, below .08 a satisfactory fit and values greater than .1 should lead to model rejection (Browne & Cudeck, 1993). For CFI and TLI, values greater than .90 indicate a good fit (Byrne, 2010). In addition, to compare the different models (M1 vs. M4), we used Akeike's Information Criterion (AIC). For AIC, smaller values represent a better model fit.

Finally, we performed a bootstrap on 2000 subsamples from the original data using the ML estimator with bias-corrected 95% confidence intervals for each of the parameter bootstrap estimates to test whether the pathways between the independent variables and the outcome variable via the mediator did, in fact, represent significant mediated relationships (see e.g. Hayes, 2009).

Results

Descriptive statistics

The means, standard deviations and correlations of the study variables are presented in Table 1. All correlations between the study variables were positive and therefore in the expected direction.

Measurement model

Before testing the hypothesized structural model, we estimated the so-called measurement model for all observed and unobserved variables simultaneously. The measurement model tests the measurement assumptions, relating the observed variables of the structural equation model to the latent factors while latent variables of the model are treated as common factors with no constraints on the correlations among the factors (Mulaik & James, 1995). Table 2 shows that the measurement model (MM) produced an acceptable fit to the data. The value of RMSEA fell below the limit of .08, whereas CFI and TLI exceeded the criterion of .90. All factor loadings of the latent variables exceeded the conventional minimum of .40, and the modification indices (MIs) did not indicate any cross-loadings or other needs for re-specifications in the model.

Testing the hypothesized model

Table 2 shows the fit indices and chi-square difference tests of the five models that were tested. The hypothesized mediation model (M1) fitted well to the data and significantly better than the direct effects model (M3) in which job resources and self-esteem at T1 only directly predicted work ability at T2 ($\Delta\chi^2 = 35.66$, $df = 1$, $p < .001$). However, there was no statistically significant difference between the hypothesized M1 and the partial mediation model (M2) in which job resources and self-esteem at T1 both directly, and

Table 2. Fit statistics for the study models and structural model comparison ($N = 403$).

Model	Description	χ^2	df	CFI	TLI	RMSEA	AIC	Model comparisons	$\Delta\chi^2$	Δdf
MM	Measurement model	71.91	27	.97	.94	.064	147.91			
M1	Hypothesized mediation model	76.33	29	.97	.94	.064	148.33			
M2	Partial mediation model	71.91	27	.97	.94	.064	147.91	M1 vs. M2	4.42 ns	2
M3	Direct effects model	111.99	30	.95	.90	.082	181.99	M1 vs. M3	35.66***	1
M4	Alternative direct effects model	94.92	28	.96	.91	.077	168.92	M1 vs. M4	18.59***	1
M5	Alternative model	80.97	30	.97	.94	.065	150.97	M1 vs. M5	4.64*	1

Notes: χ^2 = chi-square; df = degrees of freedom; CFI = Comparative Fit Index; TLI = Tucker-Lewis Index; RMSEA = Root Mean Square Error of Approximation; AIC = Akaike's Information Criterion; $\Delta\chi^2$ = chi-square difference; Δdf = degrees of freedom difference.
*$p < .05$; ***$p < .001$.

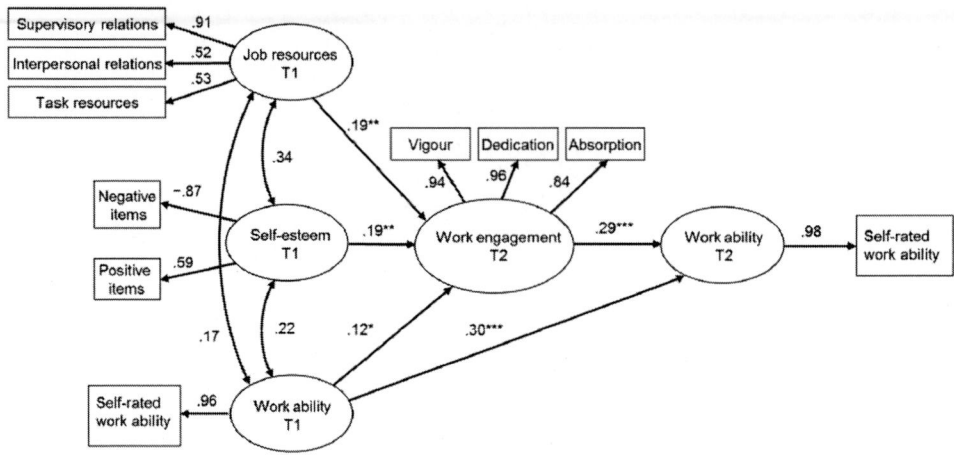

Figure 2.   Final model of the mediating role of work engagement between job resources, self-esteem and work ability (N = 403). The circles represent unobserved latent factors (e.g. work ability), and squares observed variables (e.g. self-rated work ability).
Note: ***p < .001; **p < .01; *p < .05.

indirectly via engagement, predicted work ability at T2 (χ^2 = 4.42, Δdf = 2; ns). Since M2 did not improve the model fit compared with M1, the more parsimonious M1 was considered the better model.

To compare M1 with the competing non-nested and non-mediated M4 in which job resources, self-esteem and work ability at T1 only directly predicted both engagement and work ability at T2, we used Akaike's Information Criterion (AIC). AIC was larger for M4 (AIC = 168.92), thus representing a better fit for M1 (AIC = 148.33). Finally, we tested M1 against a similar model (M5), but without the path from work ability at T1 to engagement at T2. M1 fitted significantly better to the data than M5 (χ^2 = 4.64, Δdf = 1; p < .05), thus indicating the robustness of our finding that engagement partially mediates the impact of work ability at T1 on work ability at T2.

In the best-fitting model, M1 (see Figure 2), both job resources at T1 (β = .19, p < .01) and self-esteem at T1 (β = .19, p < .01) were positively related to work engagement at T2. Furthermore, work engagement at T2 was positively related to work ability at T2 (β = .29, p < .001). Work ability at T1 also predicted work ability at T2 10 years later (β = .30, p < .001), as well as work engagement at T2 (β = .12, p < .05). The hypothesized model explained 12% of the variance in work engagement at T2 and 21% of the variance in work ability at T2.

Finally, we used bootstrapping to test whether job resources, self-esteem and work ability at T1 yielded an indirect effect via work engagement on work ability at T2. Table 3 shows that all indirect effects were confirmed, thus supporting the mediating role of work engagement between the three T1 predictors (job resources, self-esteem and work ability) and work ability at T2.

Taken together, Hypotheses 1 and 2 on the mediating role of work engagement between job resources and work ability, and between self-esteem and work ability, respectively, were supported. In addition, Hypotheses 3 regarding the partial mediation of work engagement was also supported, as work ability at T1 had an indirect effect on work ability at T2, via work engagement.

Table 3. Indirect pathways using bootstrapping.

	Bootstrapping		BC 95% CI		
	Estimate	*SE*	Lower	Upper	*p*
Indirect effect x → m → y					
Job resources → work engagement → work ability T2	.062	.027	.018	.127	.001
Self-esteem → work engagement → work ability T2	.056	.027	.014	.124	.010
Work ability T1 → work engagement → work ability T2	.036	.019	.004	.081	.037

Note: Standardized coefficients. *SE* = standard error; BC = bias corrected; CI = confidence interval.

Discussion

The purpose of this study was to expand on previous studies on job and personal resources, work engagement and work ability within the Job Demands-Resources framework and using COR theory (Hobfoll, 1989, 2001), BaB theory (Fredrickson, 2001) and self-enhancement theory (Jones, 1973) as additional conceptual frameworks. More specifically, the impact of various kinds of resources (i.e. job, personal and health-related resources) on future work ability via work engagement was studied and all our study hypotheses were supported.

By using a 10-year longitudinal design, our results contribute to the literature in at least three ways. First, we found that work engagement fully mediated the relationship between job resources and self-esteem on work ability 10 years later, thus expanding the potential outcomes of the motivational process included in the JD-R model (Hypotheses 1 and 2, respectively). Second, our findings showed that work engagement and work ability were positively associated. This finding contributes significantly to the work ability literature, which has mainly focused on individual lifestyle- and work-related risk factors, and so far ignored the importance of motivational factors in explaining work ability (Ilmarinen, 2009). Third, our results show that work ability may be an important health-related resource itself, as it predicts work engagement 10 years later, which, in its turn, is positively associated with concurrent work ability (Hypothesis 3). The current study is one of the first on work ability that focuses not only on the antecedents of work ability but also on the positive consequences it may have (see also Feldt et al., 2009).

Job and personal resources and work ability

Our study showed that job and personal resources (self-esteem) may lead not only to positive organizational outcomes, such as better job performance (Salanova et al., 2005) and organizational commitment (Hakanen, Schaufeli et al., 2008), but also to improved work ability. Job resources had motivational potential as they were related to future work engagement, and consequently to work ability. Thus, jobs characterized by supportive conditions such as autonomous tasks, positive interactions between co-workers and support and positive feedback from one's supervisor, may foster flourishing and engaged employees who enjoy good work ability. These results support SDT (Deci & Ryan, 2000), which highlights the importance of social-contextual conditions that either enhance or hinder motivation at work. In our study, we measured task resources (autonomy, skill variety and feedback) and social resources (interpersonal and supervisory relations). Autonomy was related to participants' ability to exert control over their tasks; competence was related to their opportunities to use their skills and feedback; and supervisory relations and interpersonal relations were related to the relatedness need of the SDT, all of which are related to work engagement.

In addition, our results indicated that self-esteem as a personal resource plays a significant role in shaping work engagement, and via engagement also work ability in the long term, even when the impacts of baseline work ability and job resources are controlled for. In other words, the way in which people evaluate themselves affects how engaged they are, and how they assess their work ability. Thus, if a worker has a favourable attitude towards himself, considers himself worthy and respects himself, he is more likely to be enthusiastic about his work, and is more willing to put his energy into work than a colleague with low self-esteem. Moreover, he also has better work ability than his co-worker who evaluates himself or his job more negatively. As such, our results are consistent with the basic assumption of the JD-R model that highlights the relationships between personal resources, work engagement and positive work-related outcomes. In a similar vein, our results support the self-enhancement theory (Jones, 1973) that highlights the importance of self-esteem as a personal resource in promoting well-being. Our results tentatively support the COR theory's assumption of *resources caravans* (Hobfoll, 2001), that is, increasing resources (i.e. job resources and self-esteem) tend to generate new resources (i.e. work engagement and work ability), and thus form resource caravans.

The mediating role of work engagement between resources and work ability

Following the BaB theory of positive emotions (Fredrickson, 2001), we also examined the mediating role of work engagement between job and personal resources, and future work ability. It appeared, as expected, that the effects of job resources and self-esteem on work ability 10 years later were fully mediated by work engagement after controlling for baseline work ability. More specifically, increases in job resources and self-esteem at T1 were related to an increase in work engagement at T2, which, in its turn, was positively related to work ability at T2. In addition, it is noteworthy that work ability at T1 predicted work ability at T2 not only directly but also indirectly, via work engagement. Thus, our results show that work ability can be considered a health-related resource that may have beneficial effects on employee well-being also in the long term. More precisely, employees' work ability may function as a health-related resource that builds engage-ment, which, in its turn, may affect work ability positively, thus supporting BaB theory. It was not possible in the present study to directly test the positive gain cycle hypothesis between work engagement and work ability as suggested by both BaB theory and COR theory because work engagement was not measured at both time points (see also Salanova, Schaufeli, Xanthopoulou, & Bakker, 2010). However, our results suggest the possibility of such positive reciprocal relationships.

Limitations

Our study has some limitations that should be noted. First, it was based on self-report measures, which may cause systematic measurement errors (common method variance). However, we conducted Harman's single factor test as suggested by Podsakoff, MacKenzie, Lee, and Podsakoff (2003). The test showed that common method variance did not pose a problem because the one-factor solution did not account for the majority of the covariance among the measures. Moreover, the longitudinal design used in the current study may diminish the risk of common method bias (Doty & Glick, 1998). Nevertheless, future research would benefit from applying more objective indicators of job resources, and particularly of work ability.

Second, as we only studied job and personal resources at T1 and work engagement at T2, no causal relationship between, for example, work engagement and work ability could be determined. However, as the competing model, in which work engagement and work ability at T2 were parallel dependent variables, fitted less well than the hypothesized model, we may conclude that our model with work engagement as a mediator is a plausible one. Nevertheless, future research should investigate the effect of (and possible reciprocal relationships between) work engagement on work ability, as well as a full panel design including job and personal resources measured at all study points.

Third, the 10-year time lag used in our study may not be optimal for testing the model, as other processes such as organizational changes may have influenced the effect of independent variables on the outcomes. In general, such long time lags may lead to an underestimation of the true causal relationship between study variables (Zapf, Dormann, & Frese, 1996). However, despite the changes in the organizational structure in Finnish fire departments, the work environments and colleagues for the most part remained the same. Related to the third limitation, the effect sizes were small, albeit significant. However, the significant relationships between the study variables even over the 10-year time lag are, in fact, indicative of the robustness of the findings. In addition, even relatively small effect sizes may be salient in predicting health and well-being of employees (Ford, Woolridge, Vipanchi, Kakar, & Strahan, 2014). Nevertheless, in future studies, the research model should be tested using a shorter time lag, a full panel design and with a larger sample size, as suggested by Ford et al. (2014).

Fourth, the rather high number of dropouts may be considered a limitation. However, the differences between participants and dropouts were either non-significant or minimal. In addition, it can be expected that for the most part dropout was due to retirement because of the low retirement age among Finnish firefighters (i.e. 55 years). A stepwise increase in actual retirement age has only recently occurred in Finland; however, early retirement schemes and personal retirement arrangements (under 55 years of age) are still possible routes for retirement. Therefore, the dropout from the sample can be regarded as normal and not causing any particular bias to the results.

Finally, our study focused on only one profession: firefighters. Although some caution is needed in interpreting our results, we believe that they can be extended to other occupational sectors. First, similar evidence exists of the positive impact of work engagement on various occupational sectors and countries (e.g. Hakanen et al., 2006). Second, as job and personal resources positively affected work ability via work engagement even in a highly physically demanding job, i.e. firefighting, we assume that the same effects are also likely to be found in other occupational sectors. However, this remains to be tested.

Conclusions

Our 10-year longitudinal study showed the existence of a health-related mechanism in the motivational process of the JD-R model. Both job resources and personal resources were related to future work engagement, which, in its turn was related to work ability. Moreover, we found that work engagement partially mediated the effect of baseline work ability on work ability 10 years later. As such, our findings contribute to the work ability literature, which has mostly neglected its motivational aspects. Our results indicate that work engagement, supported by resourceful jobs and positive self-esteem, plays an important role in maintaining and promoting work ability, and consequently, possibly also in decreasing employees' intentions towards early retirement.

Funding

This study was supported by grants from the Fire Protection Fund, Finland, and the Emergency Services College, Kuopio, Finland.

References

Ahlstrom, L., Grimby-Ekman, A., Hagberg, M., & Dellve, L. (2010). The work ability index and single-item question: Associations with sick leave, symptoms, and health – a prospective study of women on long-term sick leave. *Scandinavian Journal of Work, Environment & Health*, *36*, 404–412.

Airila, A., Hakanen, J., Punakallio, A., Lusa, S., & Luukkonen, R. (2012). Is work engagement related to work ability beyond working conditions and lifestyle factors? *International Archives of Occupational and Environmental Health*, *85*, 915–925.

Alarcon, G., Eschleman, K. J., & Bowling, N. A. (2009). Relationships between personality variables and burnout: A meta-analysis. *Work & Stress*, *23*, 244–263.

Arbuckle, J. L. (2009). *Amos 18 user's guide*. Chicago, IL: Amos Development Corporation.

Bakker, A., & Demerouti, E. (2007). The job demands-resources model: State of the art. *Journal of Managerial Psychology*, *22*, 309–328.

Baumeister, R. F., Campbell, J. D., Krueger, J. I., & Vohs, K. D. (2003). Does high self-esteem cause better performance, interpersonal success, happiness, or healthier lifestyles? *Psychological Science in the Public Interest*, *4*, 1–44.

Browne, M. W., & Cudeck, R. (1993). Alternative ways of assessing model fit. In J. S. Long (Ed.), *Testing structural equation models* (pp. 136–162). Newbury Park, NJ: Sage.

Byrne, B. M. (2010). *Structural equation modeling with AMOS. Basic concepts, applications, and programming* (2nd ed.). New York, NY: Routledge.

Deci, E. L., & Ryan, R. M. (2000). The "what" and "why" of goal pursuits: Human needs and the self-determination of behavior. *Psychological Inquiry*, *11*, 227–268.

Demerouti, E., Bakker, A. B., Nachreiner, F., & Schaufeli, W. B. (2001). The job demands-resources model of burnout. *Journal of Applied Psychology*, *86*, 499–512.

Doty, H. D., & Glick, W. H. (1998). Common methods bias: Does common methods variance really bias results? *Organizational Research Methods*, *1*, 374–406.

Elo, A.-L., Leppänen, A., Lindström, K., & Ropponen, T. (1992). *OSQ Occupational stress questionnaire: User's instructions*. Helsinki: Institute of Occupational Health.

Feldt, T., Hyvönen, K., Mäkikangas, A., Kinnunen, U., & Kokko, K. (2009). Development trajectories of Finnish managers' work ability over a 10-year follow-up period. *Scandinavian Journal of Work, Environment & Health*, *35*, 37–47.

Ford, M. T., Woolridge, J. D., Vipanchi, M., Kakar, U. M., & Strahan, S. R. (2014). How do occupational stressor-strain effects vary with time? A review and meta-analysis of the relevance of time lags in longitudinal studies. *Work & Stress*, *28*, 9–30.

Fredrickson, B. L. (2001). The role of positive emotions in positive psychology. The broaden-and-build theory of positive emotions. *American Psychologist*, *56*, 218–226.

Hakanen, J. J., Bakker, A. B., & Jokisaari, M. (2011). A 35-year follow-up study on burnout among Finnish employees. *Journal of Occupational Health Psychology*, *16*, 345–360.

Hakanen, J. J., Bakker, A. B., & Schaufeli, W. B. (2006). Burnout and work engagement among teachers. *Journal of School Psychology*, *43*, 495–513.

Hakanen, J. J., Peeters, M., & Perhoniemi, R. (2011). Enrichment processes and gain spirals at work and at home: A three-year cross-lagged panel study. *Journal of Occupational and Organizational Psychology, 84*, 8–30.

Hakanen, J., Perhoniemi, R., & Toppinen-Tanner, S. (2008). Positive gain spirals at work: From job resources to work engagement, personal initiative and work-unit innovativeness. *Journal of Vocational Behavior, 73*, 78–91.

Hakanen, J. J., & Roodt, G. (2010). Using the job demands-resources model to predict work engagement: Analysing the conceptual model. In A. B. Bakker & M. P. Leiter (Eds.), *Work engagement: A handbook of essential theory and research* (pp. 85–101). New York, NY: Psychology Press.

Hakanen, J. J., & Schaufeli, W. B. (2012). Do burnout and work engagement predict depressive symptoms and life satisfaction? A three-wave seven-year prospective study. *Journal of Affective Disorders, 141*, 415–424.

Hakanen, J. J., Schaufeli, W. B., & Ahola, K. (2008). The job demands-resources model: A three-year cross-lagged study of burnout, depression, commitment, and work engagement. *Work & Stress, 22*, 224–241.

Haslam, C., & Mallon, K. (2003). A preliminary investigation of post-traumatic stress symptoms among firefighters. *Work & Stress, 17*, 277–285.

Hayes, A. F. (2009). Beyond Baron and Kenny: Statistical mediation analysis in the new millennium. *Communication Monographs, 76*, 408–420.

Hobfoll, S. E. (1989). Conservation of resources. A new attempt at conceptualizing stress. *American Psychologist, 44*, 513–524.

Hobfoll, S. E. (2001). The influence of culture, community, and the nested-self in the stress process: Advancing conservation of resources theory. *Applied Psychology: An International Review, 50*, 337–421.

Hobfoll, S. E., Johnson, R. J., Ennis, N., & Jackson, A. P. (2003). Resource loss, resource gain, and emotional outcomes among inner city women. *Journal of Personality and Social Psychology, 84*, 632–643.

Ilmarinen, J. (2009). Work ability – A comprehensive concept for occupational health research and prevention. *Scandinavian Journal of Work, Environment & Health, 35*, 1–5.

Janssen, P. P. M., Schaufeli, W. B., & Houkes, I. (1999). Work-related and individual determinants of the three burnout dimensions. *Work & Stress, 13*, 74–86.

Jones, S. C. (1973). Self and interpersonal evaluations: Esteem theories versus consistency theories. *Psychological Bulletin, 79*, 185–199.

Kalimo, R., Pahkin, K., Mutanen, P., & Toppinen-Tanner, S. (2003). Staying well or burning out at work: Work characteristics and personal resources as long-term predictors. *Work & Stress, 17*, 109–122.

Kauppinen, T., Hanhela, R., Kandolin, I., Karjalainen, A., Kasvio, A., Perkiö-Mäkelä, M., … Viluksela, M. (Eds.). (2010). *Työ ja terveys Suomessa* [Work and Health in Finland]. Helsinki: Työterveyslaitos.

Langelaan, S., Bakker, A. B., Schaufeli, W. B., Van Rhenen, W., & Van Doornen, L. J. P. (2006). Do burned-out and work-engaged employees differ in the functioning of the hypothalamic-pituitary-adrenal axis. *Scandinavian Journal of Work, Environment & Health, 32*, 339–348.

Lusa, S., Punakallio, A., & Luukkonen, R. (2011). Factors predicting perceived work ability of Finnish firefighters. In C-H. Nygård, M. Savinainen, T. Kirsi, & K. Lumme-Sandt (Eds.), *Age management during the life course. Proceedings of the 4th symposium on work ability* (pp. 161–169). Tampere: Tampere University Press.

Lusa, S., Punakallio, A., Luukkonen, R., & Louhevaara, V. (2006). Factors associated with changes in perceived strain at work among fire-fighters: a 3-year follow-up study. *International Archives of Occupational and Environmental Health, 79*, 419–426.

Marsh, H. W. (1996). Positive and negative global self-esteem: A substantively meaningful distinction or artifactors? *Journal of Personality and Social Psychology, 70*, 810–919.

Mitani, S., Fujita, M., Nakata, K., & Shirakawa, T. (2006). Impact of post-traumatic stress disorder and job-related stress on burnout: A study of fire service workers. *The Journal of Emergency Medicine, 31*, 7–11.

Mulaik, S., & James, L. (1995). Objectivity and reasoning in science and structural equation modeling. In R. Hoyle (Ed.), *Structural equation modeling: Concepts, issues, and applications* (pp. 118–137). Thousand Oaks, CA: Sage.

Ouweneel, E., Le Blanc, P., Schaufeli, W. B., & Van Wijhe, C. (2012). Good morning, good day: A diary study on positive emotions, hope, and work engagement. *Human Relations, 65,* 1129–1154.

Parzefall, M.-R., & Hakanen, J. (2010). Psychological contract and its motivational and health-enhancing properties. *Journal of Managerial Psychology, 25,* 4–21.

Podsakoff, P. M., MacKenzie, S. B., Lee, J., & Podsakoff, N. P. (2003). Common method biases in behavioral research: A critical review of the literature and recommended remedies. *Journal of Applied Psychology, 88,* 879–903.

Rosenberg, M. (1965). *Society and the adolescent self-image.* Princeton, NJ: Princeton University Press.

Rosenberg, M., Schooler, C., Schoenbach, C., & Rosenberg, F. (1995). Global self-esteem and specific self-esteem: Different concepts, different outcomes. *American Sociological Review, 60,* 141–156.

Saijo, Y., Ueno, T., & Hashimoto, Y. (2007). Job stress and depressive symptoms among Japanese fire fighters. *American Journal of Industrial Medicine, 50,* 470–480.

Salanova, M., Agut, S., & Peiró, J. M. (2005). Linking organizational resources and work engagement to employee performance and customer loyalty: The mediation of service climate. *Journal of Applied Psychology, 90,* 1217–1227.

Salanova, M., Schaufeli, W. B., Xanthopoulou, D., & Bakker, A. B. (2010). The gain spiral of resources and work engagement: Sustaining a positive worklife. In A. B. Bakker & M. P. Leiter (Eds.), *Work engagement: A handbook of essential theory and research* (pp. 118–131). New York, NY: Psychology Press.

Salmela-Aro, K., & Nurmi, J.-E. (2007). Self-esteem during university studies predicts career characteristics 10 years later. *Journal of Vocational Behavior, 70,* 463–477.

Schaufeli, W. B., Bakker, A. B., & Salanova, M. (2006). The measurement of work engagement with a short questionnaire. A cross-national study. *Educational and Psychological Measurement, 66,* 701–716.

Schaufeli, W., Salanova, M., González-Roma, V., & Bakker, A. B. (2002). The measurement of engagement and burnout: A two sample confirmatory factor analytic approach. *The Journal of Happiness Studies, 3,* 71–92.

Schaufeli, W. B., & Taris, T. W. (2014). A critical review of the job Demands-resources model: Implications for improving work and health. In G. F. Bauer & O. Hämmig (Eds.), *Bridging occupational, organizational and public health* (pp. 43–68). Amsterdam: Springer.

Seitsamo, J., von Bonsdorff, M. E., Ilmarinen, J., von Bonsdorff, M. B., Nygård, C.-H., Rantanen, T., & Klockars, M. (2011). Work ability and later-life health: A 28-year longitudinal study among Finnish municipal workers. In C-H. Nygård, M. Savinainen, T. Kirsi, & K. Lumme-Sandt (Eds.), *Age management during the life course.* Proceedings of the 4th symposium on work ability (pp 391–398). Tampere: Tampere University Press.

Seppälä, P., Mauno, S., Kinnunen, M., Feldt, T., Juuti, T., Tolvanen, A., & Rusko, H. (2012). Is work engagement related to healthy cardiac autonomic activity? Evidence from a field study among Finnish women workers. *Journal of Positive Psychology, 7,* 95–106.

Tengland, P. A. (2011). The concept of work ability. *Journal of Occupational Rehabilitation, 21,* 275–285.

Tuomi, K., Ilmarinen, J., Jahkola, A., Katajarinne, L., & Tulkki, A. (1998). *Work Ability Index* (2nd revised ed.). Helsinki: Institute of Occupational Health.

Van den Berg, T. I. J., Elders, L. A. M., Zwart, B. C. H., & Burdorf, A. (2009). The effects of work-related and individual factors on the work ability index: A systematic review. *Occupational and Environmental Medicine, 66,* 211–220.

Van den Broeck, A., Vansteenkiste, M., De Witte, H., & Lens, W. (2008). Explaining the relationships between job characteristics, burnout, and engagement: The role of basic psychological need satisfaction. *Work & Stress, 22,* 277–294.

Williamson, D. L., & Carr, J. (2009). Health as a resource for everyday life: advancing the conceptualization. *Critical Public Health, 19,* 107–122.

World Health Organization (WHO). (1986). *Ottawa charter for health promotion. First international conference on health promotion.* Ottawa: Author.

Xanthopoulou, D., Bakker, A. B., Demerouti, E., & Schaufeli, W. B. (2007). The role of personal resources in the job demands-resources model. *International Journal of Stress Management, 14,* 121–141.

Xanthopoulou, D., Bakker, A. B., Demerouti, E., & Schaufeli, W. B. (2009). Reciprocal relationships between job resources, personal resources and work engagement. *Journal of Vocational Behavior, 74,* 235–244.

Zapf, D., Dormann, C., & Frese, M. (1996). Longitudinal studies in organizational stress research: A review of the literature with reference to methodological issues. *Journal of Occupational Health Psychology, 1,* 145–169.

Index